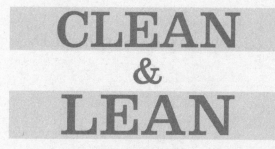

CLEAN
&
LEAN

Also by Ian K. Smith, M.D.

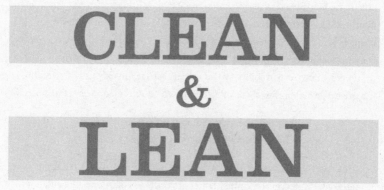

CLEAN & LEAN

30 DAYS,
30 FOODS,
A **NEW** YOU!

Ian K. Smith, M.D.

ST. MARTIN'S GRIFFIN

NEW YORK

Published in the United States by St. Martin's Griffin,
an imprint of St. Martin's Publishing Group

CLEAN & LEAN. Copyright © 2019 by Ian K. Smith, M.D. All rights reserved. Printed in the United States of America. For information, address St. Martin's Publishing Group, 120 Broadway, New York, NY 10271.

www.stmartins.com

The Library of Congress has cataloged the hardcover edition as follows:

Names: Smith, Ian, 1969– author.
Title: Clean & lean : 30 days, 30 foods, a new you! / Ian K. Smith, M.D.
Other titles: Clean and lean
Description: First edition. | New York, NY : St. Martin's Press, 2019.
Identifiers: LCCN 2019005315 | ISBN 9781250114945 (hardcover) |
    ISBN 9781250114952 (ebook)
Subjects: LCSH: Reducing diets. | Reducing diets—Recipes. | Nutrition. |
    Exercise.
Classification: LCC RM222.2 .S625 2019 | DDC 613.2/5—dc23
LC record available at https://lccn.loc.gov/2019005315

ISBN 978-1-250-22952-6 (trade paperback)

Our books may be purchased in bulk for promotional, educational, or business use. Please contact your local bookseller or the Macmillan Corporate and Premium Sales Department at 1-800-221-7945, extension 5442, or by email at MacmillanSpecialMarkets@macmillan.com.

First St. Martin's Griffin Edition: December 2019

10 9 8 7 6 5 4 3 2 1

To my brother, Michael Strahan.
Thanks for all the great memories.
Let's make a whole lot more.
Whoever thought we'd have so much fun?
See ya on the golf course!

CONTENTS

ACKNOWLEDGMENTS

I am always grateful to those who inspire and support me in my work. Since my book *SHRED: The Revolutionary Diet*, I have built a loyal and reliable following, particularly those in my robust and productive Facebook groups: SHREDDER Nation, TheClean20, and Clean & Lean. (Join us!) I learn from them as much if not more than they learn from me. They inspired me to write this book and I'm forever grateful. While there are tens of thousands in this group, and I'm forever grateful to all of them, I wanted to give a special shout-out to a few: Beverly Simon, Felicia Tate, Sandra Chiasson—my faithful and energetic admins who keep the trains running—as well as Rosemary Delarosa, Kimberly Slaughter Cunningham, and Kevin Snyder. Thank you all for inspiring me and others, and for always being there when people in the groups have questions or need encouragement. Most of all, you've led by example and that is worth a million words. You've literally changed and saved thousands of lives, and it simply doesn't get much better than that!

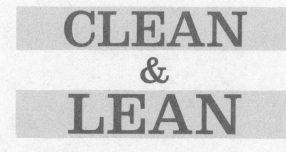

CLEAN
&
LEAN

INTRODUCTION

I have always professed that understanding nutrition and successful weight loss is a lifelong process. I continue to believe that. This is especially the case when trying to create programs that are doable, effective, scientifically based, and sustainable. Despite the numerous books I've written on weight loss and nutrition, I continue to read, research, listen, and learn. Thus, the impetus for *Clean & Lean*.

One of my faithful followers messaged me about using my most recent program, The Clean 20, with the concept of intermittent fasting. She had been doing it on her own and had found improved results, especially after hitting a plateau. At the same time, one of my best friends, Nazr Mohammed, a former NBA player, decided he wanted to try intermittent fasting in the form of time restricted eating, in which he ate only between the hours of noon and 8 p.m. He had heard of others doing this and they had found success.

I asked both of them questions and listened intently to their methods, challenges, and insights. Two very different people—a woman in her sixties on the verge of retirement and a former professional athlete who had spent the vast majority of his life training and eating for peak performance—trying a similar eating strategy. I learned a significant amount and that led me to plunge into the available research of intermittent fasting, its benefits, strategies, and effects not just on weight, but on other important health biomarkers.

Intermittent fasting, while not heavily researched in humans yet, has shown promise in animal studies and via anecdotal evidence in humans. Clean eating, the basis of my last book, *The Clean 20*, has also shown particular benefits not just on the scale (average of 10-pound weight loss in twenty days), but in lowering cholesterol levels, glucose levels, and blood pressure. So why not combine the two and see if the benefits would be synergistic? It made complete sense to do this, and from the standpoint of execution it was a strategy I felt most people would be able to follow long enough to get results and return to if they wanted to tune up their bodies at other times.

Regardless of how well created or executed, no one diet plan works for everyone. Our bodies are different in so many ways, from the way we metabolize certain foods to the way we accumulate fat and the way we lose it. But Clean & Lean is a program that I believe the vast majority of people will be able to follow to achieve measurable results. I'm trimming the fat (literally and figuratively) and getting right to the point so that this might be one of the simplest nutrition books you'll ever follow. Get ready to welcome a *new you* in thirty days!

Ian K. Smith, M.D.
April 2019

I

The PREP

1

UNDERSTANDING INTERMITTENT FASTING

The concept of intermittent fasting (IF) is not particularly new, but over the last several years it has garnered a lot of attention and new research. It is what it sounds like—periods of fasting alternating with periods of non-fasting. While the vast majority of research has been conducted in animals, there have been more human-based studies the last couple of years that have analyzed the biological and physiologic changes that occur once a person participates in an IF program.

There are two major types of IF eating schedules. The first is the 5:2 schedule, where for five days a person eats how they typically would, then for two days of the week calories are restricted to 800 or less. The one caveat is that the fasting days should not be consecutive.

The second type of eating schedule, which you will follow on Clean & Lean, is time restricted feeding (TRF). On it, food is consumed only during certain hours and there are two periods of fasting. The duration of the feeding periods can vary. Most commonly, they are 8, 10, or 12 hours in length. For example, a 16:8 strategy includes 16 hours of fasting and 8 hours of feeding; the 14:10 strategy would be 14 hours of fasting and 10 hours of feeding.

The two IF eating schedules would look something like this:

5:2 INTERMITTENT FASTING

Monday	Tuesday	Wednesday	Thursday	Friday	Saturday	Sunday
Normal eating	Normal eating	Fasting (800 calories or less)	Normal eating	Normal eating	Fasting (800 calories or less)	Normal eating

TIME RESTRICTED FEEDING (TRF)

7 A.M.	7–10 A.M.	10 A.M.–8 P.M.	8 P.M.–10 A.M.
Wake up	Fasting	Feeding	Fasting

Benefits of IF

Researchers acknowledge that while IF has been used for several years, and there have been studies performed to analyze the pros and cons of this eating strategy, much more work needs to be done to make validated, scientifically based claims. There have been, however, lots of anecdotal evidence about the effects of IF as well as animal studies and early human trials. While these observations are not always definitive and conclusive, they give us a clearer window through which we can inspect the potential benefits of this eating strategy. The evidence suggests that IF can help in weight loss, better regulate blood sugar levels, increase blood levels of human growth hormone, and induce cellular repair processes.

Potential Benefits of Intermittent Fasting

- Weight Loss
- Decreased Inflammation
- Improved Asthma-Related Symptoms
- Preserved Learning and Memory Functioning
- Decreased Belly Fat
- Reduced Insulin Resistance

Given the various research studies looking at IF, there are many theories that have been suggested as to why there might be appreciable physiological benefits. Mark Mattson, a senior investigator from the National Institute of Aging, has studied the hypothesis that during the fasting period cells are actually subjected to a mild stress. Mattson and others believe that cells react by making adaptations that increase their ability to handle this stress and possibly resist disease. It's akin to the adage, "Whatever doesn't kill you, makes you stronger." In other words, fasting deprives cells of nourishment, which is stressful. But the cells change and adapt to handle tough conditions. Scientists believe that these changes make the cells tougher and better at preventing or fighting disease.

Intermittent fasting does not mean that you can simply eat whatever you want or how much you want during feeding times and still lose weight. One of the big misconceptions held by many people is that as long as they don't violate their eating time parameters they can indulge in as many sweets, alcoholic beverages, or fried foods as they desire. Not only is this untrue, but it can potentially be very harmful to one's health and efforts at losing or maintaining a healthy weight.

Calorie consumption still matters even while employing the IF strategy. For example, whether you consume 3,700 calories within a regulated 10-hour time span or throughout the day as is typical, the basic equation of weight loss still holds. Calories in must be less than calories out in order to lose weight. The vast majority of people who are consuming 3,700 calories are not going to lose weight regardless of the number of hours it takes to consume those calories. The body must do something with the caloric energy that is consumed. If you don't burn off the calories, the body will store them in the form of fat, which will not only increase your weight but prevent you from attaining that leaner physique you're trying to achieve.

Feeding Times

There are three TRF schedules that we will focus on in this book: 16 hours of fasting with 8 hours of feeding (16:8), 14 hours of fasting with 10 hours of feeding (14:10), and 12 hours of fasting with 12 hours of feeding (12:12). If you're not sure which schedule will best fit you, try the 14:10 plan first. If it seems too difficult after a few days, then switch to the 12:12 plan. If it seems too easy, and you are up to the challenge, give the 16:8 a try. While the specific hours you choose to start and end your periods of fasting and feeding can change according to your preference, on the next page are samples of what a schedule might look like. You choose the feeding timetable that works best for you, but keep in mind that the smaller feeding window might produce better results.

16:8 FASTING/FEEDING RATIO

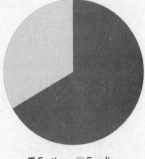

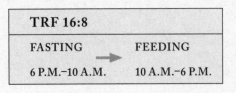

TRF 16:8	
FASTING	FEEDING
6 P.M.–10 A.M.	10 A.M.–6 P.M.

■ Fasting ■ Feeding

14:10 FASTING/FEEDING RATIO

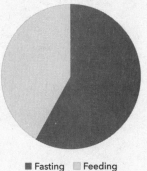

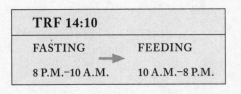

TRF 14:10	
FASTING	FEEDING
8 P.M.–10 A.M.	10 A.M.–8 P.M.

■ Fasting ■ Feeding

12:12 FASTING/FEEDING RATIO

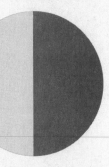

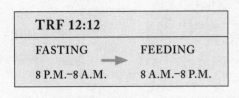

TRF 12:12	
FASTING	FEEDING
8 P.M.–8 A.M.	8 A.M.–8 P.M.

■ Fasting ■ Feeding

2

THE CLEAN & LEAN RULES

I have designed Clean & Lean to be as accessible and versatile as possible. I don't expect you to go to a grocery store and empty your bank account in order to find the items on the list. I don't expect you to be locked into your house for the next thirty days so that you are in complete control of your food environment and all the ingredients that go into your food. You will be at work or at a restaurant or in an airport, and you still need to eat and not feel like you're a criminal because you might have to slightly alter the plan. Remember, the purpose of Clean & Lean is to reintroduce your body to the wonders of clean eating and to give your organs a break from all the processed foods that dominate the choices in our stores and restaurants.

Clean food and clean recipes don't have to be boring or flavorless, despite the image conjured of plain chicken and bland raw vegetables. In fact, clean foods can be just as tasty and exciting as those processed foods that are loaded with lots of additives and artificial flavor enhancers. Spices and clean condiments can go a long way to liven up recipes and thrill your palate. We have grown so accustomed to processed foods that we need to be reacquainted with the authentic flavors of real, natural food. So take your time with the ingredients. Taste them raw or with spices—something that will happen over the next thirty days.

I don't like to use the word "rules," because the mere mention of it inspires eye-rolling and rebellion and annoyance. Most people don't like to be told what they can and can't do as well as what they can and can't eat. But in order for you to maximize your results and reset your experience for the next thirty days, I created guidelines that will give you the greatest chance of success and keep you most in line with the plan's overall mission. A plan without any rules or guidelines would be a free-for-all, and it's highly unlikely that would produce the results you're seeking.

I have learned over the years that no chapter or book can answer all of the possible questions that come up. Just when you think you've covered all the bases, someone finds a topic or angle that hasn't been addressed. I am not perfect, and this plan is not perfect. However, between the guidelines below and some common sense, the next thirty days should work well for you.

The key to success on this plan definitely lies in the departments of planning and preparation. Take a little time to think about what the next several days will look like: what meals you'll be consuming and where they'll be consumed. If you're going to be traveling, take that into account and think about what foods will most likely be available to you while on the road. Plan accordingly.

1. No soda (regular or diet)

This is the biggest NO on the plan. Despite the taste that many enjoy, soda has *absolutely* no redeeming nutritional qualities at all. Full of sugar, artificial sweeteners, additives, and other mystery chemicals, it is like drinking fizzy poison. This goes for diet soda, too, which is equally filled with artificial ingredients. If soda is something you regularly drink, just cutting it out will make you feel like a new person. I have had hundreds if not thousands of people either write to me or tell me in person how cutting soda from their diet completely turned things around for them.

2. Only freshly squeezed juice

There is a thing called natural sugar. Sugar that is found in freshly squeezed juice comes just as nature created it. Yes, it's still sugar, and yes, it still has calories, but it's what comes with the sugar that makes the difference. Natural sugar does not prevent a food or drink from being clean; rather, it's when the sugar is *added* that makes the difference. It's what I call the "sugar package." Vitamins and minerals and other phytonutrients come along with the sugar in fresh juice and are paramount at boosting our health. If you're going to consume sugar, at least get some nutritional bang for your buck. One tip is, if it's possible, get freshly squeezed juice that hasn't been completely strained of the pulp and fruit skin, which contain lots of nutrients. Be careful of the labeling. For the purposes of Clean & Lean, you should not be drinking anything from concentrate or major manufacturer brands that just say "100% juice." You should be looking for juices that are "freshly squeezed" and are labeled "no sugar added." The ingredients should only list juice from fruit or fruits and in some cases water, but nothing else.

3. Canned and frozen are allowed

These items are allowed, but they must be clean. Nothing artificial is allowed, and the foods must be packaged in water or their natural juices. Something like canned tuna in water is completely fine, as are organic frozen vegetables and fruits. With anything canned or frozen, always be mindful of the sodium content, as it tends to be high, so opt for low-sodium options. Before turning your nose at frozen produce, you should be aware that the fresh fruit and vegetables you purchase at the store might not be as fresh as they look. In fact, a lot of produce is kept in storage for weeks at a time before it's put out for retail. Some fruits and veggies can lose up to 75% of a certain nutrient after sitting in storage for a week or more; while they may look fresh externally, there's internal degradation occurring the whole time thanks to enzymes that continue to work even after the fruit or vegetable is harvested. If you're in the market for frozen produce, search for products that have been "flash frozen." This means they have been frozen very quickly after being harvested, thus preserving the field-fresh taste and ensuring peak ripeness as well as the greatest nutrient density (more nutrients for fewer calories).

4. Unlimited water

Water is one of the most magical natural health-promoting wonders on earth. It comprises up to 70% of our body, and while it doesn't contain the nutrients you find in food, it is essential for our very existence. It has no calories, helps energize muscles, keeps our skin looking good, helps our kidneys eliminate wastes, and gives a helping hand in maintaining normal bowel function. Most people don't drink enough water, but for the next thirty days you're going to find out what it feels like to really hydrate your body all the way down to the cells. Just because you drink to quench your thirst doesn't mean you're drinking enough. For the next thirty days you should be consuming between 8 and 10 cups per day. No water with artificial sweeteners or added chemicals. If you want sparkling water, that's completely fine. If you want to squeeze some fresh citrus in your water, that's fine too. Keep it natural and abundant and your body will be grateful.

5. No added sugar

While sugar is often vilified, and for good reason, it still plays an important role in our body. Glucose (sugar) is actually the number one source of energy for our brain. Glucose is important energy for our muscles and the billion cellular processes that take place in our bodies every second of the day. But we are consuming an extraordinarily dangerous amount that is taking a toll on our health. Added sugar is the biggest culprit—it's the sugar you add to your foods at the table or that manufacturers slip into their foods while cooking or processing them. For the next thirty days, we are going to free our bodies of all this extra sugar, and you will notice the difference in your energy levels, complexion, and mood. The first few days might be challenging, but your body is an extremely adaptable machine and it will reconfigure so that in short order you will no longer crave that sweet stuff.

6. No artificial sweeteners

This should go without saying, but sometimes the most obvious things still need to be said. "Artificial" is a forbidden word for the next thirty days. While these sweeteners don't have any calories, that's the end of their good attributes. Scientists have raised all kinds of concerns, from them increasing your risk for something called the metabolic syndrome to increasing your affinity for or addiction to even sweeter foods. Avoid them at all costs and make sure you read the labels carefully, as manufacturers can be very tricky when including them on the labels for their products, making them difficult to identify.

7. Dairy is allowed

Dairy has been getting beat up lately, and I think it's simply unfair. Sometimes dieting trends simply become too trendy for our own good. The wave of no-dairy sentiment is largely misplaced and for many people can be dangerous, as dairy provides nutrients that are critical to our overall health. Calcium, potassium, vitamin D, and protein are chief among these nutrients. Dairy is the primary source of calcium in our diets and is needed to build and preserve strong bones as well as teeth. Potassium is essential to life. Every time your heart beats it relies on potassium, which helps trigger the heart to pump and squeeze blood through the body. Potassium is also critical in helping our muscles move, nerves conduct electricity, kidneys filter blood, and blood vessels maintain blood pressure. Vitamin D works to maintain proper levels of phosphorous and calcium in the body: that's why it's an important component in building and maintaining healthy bones and teeth. It also plays a role in muscle function and keeping our immune system healthy. Dairy products such as yogurt, milk, and cheese (a great source of calcium, vitamin B12, and sodium) are rich in so many nutrients that make and keep us healthy. Some people may have an intolerance to lactose—the sugar found in milk and other dairy products—and need to be careful of which products they consume, but the vast majority of us don't have this issue and can benefit greatly from the rich and easy offerings of dairy.

8. Fruits and vegetables are important

You might find yourself in a situation where you can't find a food on your list because it's simply not available. Not a problem. You are allowed to eat any fruit or vegetable even if they're not on your list. You can eat them raw or cooked, but if they are going to be cooked, make sure that they are not cooked in anything but herbs and olive oil with some spices. You can add as wide a variety of fruits and vegetables as you like, even if it pushes your list beyond thirty. These power foods are the absolute essence of clean eating!

9. No MSG

Monosodium glutamate is the salt version of the amino acid glutamate. While MSG can occur naturally in foods such as tomatoes and cheeses, it is often synthesized in the laboratory for commercial reasons. This synthetic MSG is used around the world as a flavor enhancer, commonly added to canned vegetables, soups, processed meats, and Chinese food. While the FDA has classified it as a food ingredient that's "generally regarded as safe," it remains at the center of many a food controversy. There have been many anecdotal reports of reactions to MSG, including headaches, heart palpitations (rapid, fluttering heartbeat), nausea, chest pain, weakness, and sweating. If these reactions are actually due to the MSG, they have been mild and short-lived. The FDA requires that foods containing MSG list it in the ingredients label on the packaging as "monosodium glutamate."

10. Not all salad dressings are created equally

It is better to make your own salad dressing for these thirty days, something that is not very difficult to do. However, you might not always be able to make it yourself or have access to it. In the event you find yourself in a situation where you must purchase dressing, it should only be organic, with no sugar added, and no artificial ingredients. Make sure the dressing is either fat-free or low-fat, but read the label, as manufacturers tend to sneak a lot of sugar and artificial ingredients into these dressings. Try to purchase dressing that has the fewest number of ingredients possible (five or fewer). The best bet is to make your own dressing, which will take few ingredients and not much time. Try the simple recipes on pages 223 and 224 and you won't have to worry about not finding the correct dressing at the grocery store.

11. No frying

We don't want to take nature's clean, health-promoting food and ruin all of the whole goodness that it brings. Deep-frying foods does just that and is counter to our mission. Yes, fried food tastes better to some, but so do grilled, baked, and sautéed foods. When food is fried, more calories are added to it, because the food absorbs the fat of the cooking oils. It's okay to use olive oil to cook your food, as it is quite healthy and can enhance the nutritional value of your dish. However, cooking means sautéing your food or any preparation that is quick and doesn't subject or saturate the food to sustained high heat for a long period of time—that is the equivalent of frying.

12. No white flour allowed/Whole-wheat flour is allowed

Flour is a perfect example of taking something completely nutritious and health-promoting and destroying it. The whole-wheat grain kernel is typically milled or processed (refined) and broken down into tiny pieces. In most instances, the process completely separates the three main parts of the kernel (bran, germ, endosperm). In the case of white flour, the endosperm is the only part of the three that is used, while the other two are thrown away. This basically means that the body will treat white flour as a starch and it will have similar effects in the body as eating refined sugar. Whole-wheat flour recombines the germ and bran with the endosperm further along in the process. While it is not perfect, it is more nutritious and better than white flour and is allowed.

13. Condiments with caution

Ketchup, mustard, mayonnaise, and salsa are allowed, but there's a catch—the ketchup, mayonnaise, and salsa should be as clean as possible, and if you have the time, make them yourself to avoid mistakenly eating something that has been heavily processed. (See recipes, pages 221, 222, and 225.) Mayonnaise will not keep for the entire thirty days—it will last up to a week—so you will have to make it a couple of times. Mustard is more difficult to make without using processed ingredients and the finished product can taste quite different from the mustards you're accustomed to, so there is an allowance to purchase it. You can find several brands that make an organic product that doesn't use sugar or anything artificial. Just look at the label and read the ingredients to make sure the brand fits Clean & Lean guidelines. If you must purchase your condiments, make sure they have very few ingredients, no sugar added, and no synthetic additives. You won't always be able to choose the cleanest condiments due to the situation you might find yourself in, but do your best.

14. No alcohol

Alcohol is not exactly the devil, but it also is not the healthiest thing in the world. If you are trying to eat clean, you don't want to add any more stress to your liver than necessary, especially since it's already doing a Herculean job of scrubbing your blood of toxins. Yes, red wine can be healthy with its dose of the antioxidant resveratrol, but drinking too much of it and other types of alcohol can burden your body and impede it from carrying out many more important functions. But if you're still looking for that resveratrol, you have options. You can find it in grapes, peanuts, blueberries, cranberries, and pistachios. If you don't want to be a purist and *must* have alcohol, then a glass of red wine per day, or two natural, low-calorie beers every three days, won't hurt. But remember: only one glass of wine or two beers.

3

THE CLEAN & LEAN FOODS

The next thirty days will be a completely unique experience as you focus on eating foods that are clean, less processed, and abundant in nature's goodness. These health-promoting foods are also going to be tasty and fun and inspire creativity in how you cook them and assemble your daily meals. You will only need thirty foods to complete this plan, but if you find other foods that are clean and want to include them, by all means, feel free to do so as long as they follow the guidelines.

The Clean & Lean Food List that I created (starting on page 21) does not have to be your list. This is a list I've created for myself, but this is a flexible plan, so your list might look similar or drastically different. To increase the flexibility of the plan, I've created an "extended" list of foods that you can choose from to make up your Clean & Lean 30 foods. The items that are in parentheses are called "Basket Buddies," and you can choose them instead of the main item I've listed.

There is also a list of herbs and spices that you might use. This list is not meant to be comprehensive, but a good start to show you what's possible when planning the seasoning for your food. If you don't see a spice or herb you like, don't assume that it's not allowed. Remember the simple tenet: if it's natural and not processed with artificial ingredients, feel free to add it to your seasoning arsenal. Spices and herbs are miraculous at taking otherwise bland food and creating entirely new dishes.

Your Clean & Lean 30 list is your guide for the next thirty days, so don't rush when creating your list. Patiently and diligently think about the kinds of meals you want to eat over the next month, then populate the list accordingly. But remember, this list is not written in stone. Flexibility is the key to the program. If you want to add more items to your list and it means your count exceeds thirty, feel free to add them as long as they follow our clean rules of no processing or barely processed.

The Clean & Lean Food List

Avocados

Bacon (organic turkey bacon)*

Beef (organic or 100% grass fed with no hormones)*

Berries (*Basket Buddies: apples, pears, mangos, bananas, watermelon, honeydew melon, cantaloupe, oranges, grapefruit*)

Brown rice (*Basket Buddies: wild rice, red rice, basmati rice*)*

Cheese

Chicken

Chickpeas (*Basket Buddies: black beans, red beans, cannellini beans, pinto beans, lima beans, black-eyed peas, fresh peas*)

Duck*

Eggs

Kale (*Basket Buddies: arugula, bok choy, Brussels sprouts, cabbage, cauliflower, collard greens, spinach, Swiss chard, watercress*)

Lemons (*Basket Buddies: limes, grapefruit*)

Lentils

Nuts (*Basket Buddies: sunflower seeds, pumpkin seeds, chia seeds, hemp seeds, flax seeds*)

Oatmeal (*Basket Buddy: grits*)

Onions*

Pizza (made with whole-wheat or whole-grain flour and organic cheese)*

Pork chops (certified USDA organic)*

Seafood (cod, crab, halibut, lobster, oysters, salmon, sea bass, shrimp, tuna)

Squash (*Basket Buddies: broccoli, carrots, cucumbers, eggplant, parsnips, zucchini*)

Sushi*

Sweet potatoes (*Basket Buddy: corn*)

Tomatoes

Tortillas (organic, corn or 100% whole wheat or whole-grain)*

Turkey

Quinoa (*Basket Buddies: barley, millet, farro, whole-wheat or whole-grain couscous, tempeh*)

Veal*

100% whole-wheat or whole-grain bread (*Basket Buddies: Ezekiel bread, sprouted whole-grain bread*)

Whole-wheat or whole-grain pasta

Whole-wheat flour (*Basket Buddy: white whole-wheat flour*)*

Yogurt (*Basket Buddy: cottage cheese*)

These items are new additions to the previous Clean 20 list.

Spices, Herbs, and Others

Ajwain

Allspice

Almond meal

Anise seed

Asafoetida

Balsamic vinegar (*Basket Buddies: apple cider vinegar, rice vinegar, white wine vinegar*)

Basil

Bay leaves

Caraway seed

Cardamom

Celery flakes

Chervil

Chia seed

Chiles

Chives

Cilantro

Cinnamon

Cloves

Coriander

Cumin

Curry leaves

Dill

Extra-virgin olive oil (*Basket Buddies: avocado oil, grapeseed oil, sesame oil*)

Fennel

Fenugreek

Garlic

Ginger

Granola (organic, no preservatives or artificial ingredients, no sugar added)

Green tea (*Basket Buddies: other herbal teas that don't have any artificial ingredients*)

Honey (organic or raw)

Horseradish powder

Juniper berries

Lavender

Lemongrass

Marinara sauce (organic, low-sodium, no sugar added)

Marjoram

Mayonnaise (organic)

Milk (organic, unsweetened, fat-free or low-fat or 1%, 2%, almond, coconut, soy)

Mint

Mustard seeds

Nutmeg

Onion powder

Oregano

Paprika

Parsley

Peanut butter (organic; *Basket Buddies: almond nut butter, cashew nut butter, sunflower seed butter*)

Pepper

Poppy seeds

Rosemary

Saffron

Sage

Salt

Savory (summer or winter)

Sesame

Soy sauce (organic)

Sumac

Tarragon

Thyme

Turmeric

Vanilla

II

The PLAN

4

CLEAN & LEAN
DAILY PLAN

There will be a Clean & Lean meal plan and exercise plan that you will follow for the next thirty days. You first need to establish if you're a beginner, intermediate, or advanced exerciser. This will determine which track you will follow for the workouts. In the exercise section of the book the workouts are divided into those three levels, so when your daily plan calls for you to do a particular workout, please refer to your section of the exercise portion to see what your exercises will be for that day. If you are feeling ambitious and you think you can move up to the next level, by all means do so, but be safe and make sure you understand how to do the moves.

If you want to be a strict purist for the next thirty days, by all means follow the plan as written. This would also mean abstaining from alcohol. If you want to have some flexibility, incorporate that into your plan, but be wise and realize that your results can ultimately be impacted depending on how widely you stray or deviate from the template. There are some recipes from "Condiments" in the back of the book as well as a snacks section that you can use. If you don't want to choose the snacks from the daily meal-plan suggestions, feel free to choose from the list of snacks, beginning on page 216. If you want to improvise a little, feel free to do so, but remember the basic tenets of eating clean.

You are in charge of deciding which feeding schedule you want to follow. If you want to change the schedule after a week or two weeks, feel free to do so, but make sure you change at the beginning of the week and not in the middle. It would be a big mistake to think that you can eat as much as you want as long as you stay within the feeding schedule. Intermittent fasting can be effective, but it is rendered ineffective if you overindulge in foods that are going to add a lot of calories and processed ingredients to your daily consumption. Most important, pay attention to how you feel the next thirty days, keep track of what works and what doesn't, learn as much as you can about yourself, and, by all means, have some fun!

DAY 1

"A transformation is not a sprint, rather it's a marathon."

This is the beginning of a *new you!* Take a deep breath and relax. Allow your mind to channel positive thoughts and remind yourself that this is a journey of self-discovery, not a competition. Be patient and confident that you have what it takes to undergo this transformation. It's important to be realistic right from the beginning. Too often people set goals that are unrealistic, and then when they don't reach these goals, they get discouraged and incorrectly believe that they've failed or that the plan has failed them. You will find the most fulfilling success if you start with your mind in the right place and keep it there over the next thirty days. While tangible goals such as weight loss, muscle strengthening, and body sculpting are important, so is the goal of making sustainable lifestyle changes that will keep you feeling healthy and fit. The work you do today and over the course of the rest of the plan will put you in a prime position to live your best life unapologetically.

Meal 1 (choose 1 of the following):

- 2 eggs scrambled in a teaspoon of extra-virgin olive oil or an omelet with diced veggies; side of fruit (berries, banana, apple, melon)
- 1 cup cooked oatmeal with diced fruit and ½ teaspoon organic raw honey and cinnamon (if desired)

Meal 2 (choose 1 of the following):

- Turkey sandwich on 100% whole-wheat or whole-grain bread with 5 ounces turkey, with the option of 1 ounce cheese, plus tomato, lettuce, and organic mustard or clean mayo (see page 222), and serving of raw or cooked vegetables
- Large green garden salad with 2 tablespoons clean salad dressing (see recipes, pages 223–224) (3 to 5 ounces sliced chicken breast or fish optional)

Meal 3 (choose 1 of the following):

- 6 ounces grilled or baked skinless chicken breast with spinach and carrots (or two other vegetables of your choosing)
- 1 cup whole-wheat or whole-grain pasta with cooked vegetables and 3 to 5 ounces diced chicken

Snacks (choose 3 snacks from below and eat them whenever you want during your feeding window):

- Kale chips (½ cup raw kale, stems removed, baked with 1 teaspoon olive oil at 400°F until crisp)
- 1 cup fresh berries
- 20 raw almonds
- 15 walnuts
- ½ grapefruit
- ½ cup sunflower seeds
- 1 large apple, sliced, sprinkled with cinnamon
- Frozen banana slices
- 8 to 10 green or black olives
- ¼ cup wasabi peas

Work It Out!

> ### *Patience Is a Virtue*
>
> It's a popular position to want fast results when participating in a transformative fitness program. Once you make the decision to change your lifestyle and adopt new behaviors, it's understandable that you want these changes to yield results as quickly as possible. But you must be realistic and patient. Just like the expression "Rome was not built in a day," so it goes for your transformation. It takes time to see wholesale changes, so don't obsess on a scale or in a mirror. In fact, it's a lot more likely that someone else will notice physical changes before you do. Stick to the program and remain confident that if you do the right things the right way, change is on the way!

Beginner: Workout #1 (page 133)

Intermediate: Workout #1 (page 143)

Advanced: Workout #1 (page 153)

THE MORE YOU KNOW!

CALCIUM

The most abundant mineral in the body, it makes bones and teeth, and helps with muscle contraction and relaxation, nerve function, blood clotting, and blood pressure maintenance.

cont.

RECOMMENDED DIETARY ALLOWANCE

	Male	Female	Pregnant	Lactating
19–50 years	1,000 mg	1,000 mg	1,000 mg	1,000 mg
51–70 years	1,000 mg	1,200 mg		
71+ years	1,200 mg	1,200 mg		

DAY 2

*"Winning the small battles is ultimately
what will help you win the war."*

Congrats on reaching Day 2! Getting to this point for
many is a big deal, and there's no reason not to be excited about it.
Remember that while we're often looking for dramatic results as
quickly as possible, the small changes build the foundation for a
sustainable transformation. Results don't just flash across the LED
screen of a scale, but can be found in other areas including will-
power, making smarter decisions, and being resilient when things
aren't going so well. These are called non-scale victories (NSV) and
they are critical for overall success. Maybe you've never been
able to work out two days in a row or you resisted the urge to park
near the entrance of a building and chose a spot at the back of the
lot that will make your walk longer than normal. Learn how to
applaud even the small victories, as they are tangible reminders
that you're making changes, regardless of how small they may
be, that will move you closer to your larger goals.

Meal 1 (choose 1 of the following):

- 1 protein shake (350 calories or less)
- 1 fruit smoothie (350 calories or less)
- 1 grilled cheese sandwich made with 100% whole-wheat
  or whole-grain bread and organic cheese

Meal 2 (choose 1 of the following):

- Tuna salad sandwich on 100% whole-wheat or whole-grain bread (mix ½ can tuna, 1 teaspoon clean mayonnaise [see recipe, page 222], 1 teaspoon low-fat or fat-free organic Greek yogurt, diced celery, diced sweet pickle) with 2 servings of vegetables
- Avocado sandwich with 2 slices 100% whole-wheat or whole-grain bread, ¼ mashed avocado, 1 ounce organic cheese, 2 tomato slices

Meal 3 (choose 1 of the following):

- 5-ounce veggie burger on 100% whole-wheat or whole-grain bun with lettuce, tomato, and onion with a medium green garden salad
- 5-ounce turkey burger on 100% whole-wheat or whole-grain bun with lettuce, tomato, and onion with a medium green garden salad
- 5-ounce chicken burger on 100% whole-wheat or whole-grain bun with lettuce, tomato, and onion with a medium green garden salad

Snacks (choose 3 snacks from below and eat them whenever you want during your feeding window):

- 1 large apple or orange or banana
- 2 small peaches
- 3 cups plain air-popped popcorn (light seasoning)
- 1 cup mixed fruit salad
- ⅔ cup raw veggies with guacamole
- 15 frozen grapes
- ¼ cup mushrooms marinated in extra-virgin olive oil, salt, and pepper

- 4 clean turkey meatballs 1 inch in diameter (mix 1 pound lean ground turkey, 2 eggs, 2 cloves minced garlic, ¼ cup chopped onion, ¼ teaspoon salt, ½ teaspoon black pepper, ½ teaspoon dried oregano, ½ cup 100% whole-wheat or whole-grain bread crumbs, 1 teaspoon extra-virgin olive oil)
- ¼ cup baked apple chips
- 8 olives stuffed with 1 tablespoon feta or blue cheese

Work It Out!

Buddy Up

Find a friend either in your neighborhood, work, church, or online who will be your workout buddy. This is a person who will encourage and support you. It's ideal if they too will be working out alongside you, but if that's not possible, you can still benefit from a workout buddy who is not geographically near you. Discuss your concerns and excitement and accomplishments with your buddy. When you are down, ask them to lift you up, and vice versa. Regardless of how committed you might be to the program, having someone else in the trenches with you can help you stay focused and even have fun at times when it doesn't seem like joy is still possible.

Beginner: Workout #1 (page 133)

Intermediate: Workout #1 (page 143)

Advanced: Workout #1 (page 153)

THE MORE YOU KNOW!

COPPER

This is an essential trace mineral that is necessary for survival. It can be found in all of the body's tissues. Some of its major benefits include: aids digestion and absorption, lubricates joints and organs, regulates body temperature, and plays a role in making red blood cells and maintaining nerve cells and the immune system. Copper also helps the body form collagen and absorb iron.

RECOMMENDED DIETARY ALLOWANCE

	Male	*Female*
+19 years	900 µg	900 µg

DAY 3

*"Belief in yourself is always the first ingredient
in the recipe of success."*

The force of belief is invaluable. If you don't believe in yourself or the task at hand, the chances of you succeeding are greatly diminished. There's a great saying that "people make their own luck." Part of this is believing that whatever endeavor you're undertaking, you will be able to carry it out successfully. The mind–body connection is only enhanced when you truly believe that you're capable of accomplishing a feat regardless of how difficult or unique it might be. Belief is the engine that powers and propels you to overcome odds and make dreams become a reality. Approach each day, and the challenges that arise throughout the day, with the belief that you can overcome and succeed. Too often our doubts become a self-fulfilling prophecy, because we have conditioned our minds to expect failure or fall short of our goals. Even if the task is difficult or something you've never been able to accomplish before, the right first step toward success is believing that you can do it.

Meal 1 (choose 1 of the following):

- Turkey bacon, egg, and cheese sandwich on 100% whole-wheat or whole-grain bread with side of fruit
- 1½ cups cooked oatmeal with side of fruit (honey and cinnamon allowed)
- 2 scrambled eggs with cheese and/or veggies and 1 slice 100% whole-wheat or whole-grain toast

Meal 2 (choose 1 of the following):

- Chicken or turkey sandwich on 100% whole-wheat or whole-grain bread with lettuce, tomato, cheese, and clean mayo (see recipe, page 222) or mustard with 1 serving of vegetables or a small green garden salad
- Large green garden salad (3 to 5 ounces chicken or fish optional)

Meal 3 (choose 1 of the following):

- 6 ounces grilled or baked salmon or other fish with 2 servings of vegetables
- Vegetarian plate with a combination of vegetables and legumes such as chickpeas or beans

Snacks (choose 3 snacks from below and eat them whenever you want during your feeding window):

- 2 dates stuffed with almonds (take out the pits and replace with 2 almonds)
- 3 tomato slices and fresh basil drizzled with extra-virgin olive oil
- 8 baby carrots with 2 tablespoons hummus
- 1 slice whole-wheat or whole-grain pita bread, cut into quarters, with 2 tablespoons hummus
- 10 cherries mixed with a handful of nuts (cashews, almonds, or walnuts)
- ½ cup shelled or unshelled pistachios
- ⅓ cup egg salad made with clean mayonnaise (see recipe, page 222)
- ⅔ cup cauliflower with 2 tablespoons hummus
- 1 fat-free or low-fat mozzarella cheese stick with 1 small apple
- Sliced tomatoes with a pinch of pepper and/or salt and olive oil

Work It Out!

> ### *Recover*
>
> One of the biggest mistakes that people make when exercising is not allowing their bodies time to recover. This might sound strange, but the body actually builds muscle and endurance by getting repeatedly injured. That's right, in order for the body to improve you are constantly causing minor injuries to your tissues. These are not injuries that require medical attention; rather they are microscopic injuries that the body spontaneously repairs. These repairs actually make you better than you were before the injury. It's easy to get excited when starting a new program to push yourself in hopes of getting bigger and faster results. But remember that if your body doesn't have a chance to recover, you will actually hinder growth rather than facilitate it.

Beginner: Rest

Intermediate: Rest

Advanced: Rest

THE MORE YOU KNOW!

IRON

Part of the hemoglobin molecule that carries oxygen in the blood. It supports metabolism and is necessary for growth, development, normal cellular function, and the synthesis of some hormones.

cont.

RECOMMENDED DIETARY ALLOWANCE

	Male	*Female*
19–50 years	8 mg	18 mg
51+ years	8 mg	8 mg

DAY 4

"Control your environment and control your destiny."

Set yourself up to succeed, not fail. Make sure you create an environment that will best nourish what you are trying to accomplish. For example, if you know that you struggle with sweets, don't tempt yourself by stopping by a bakery. Limit your interactions to those with people who will be supportive of your endeavors and not dismissive. Avoid those who might try to encourage you to participate in behaviors and decision making that you're trying to change. The fewer distractions you have, the greater the likelihood that you will stay on track. Preparation is one of the greatest tools you can use to accomplish your goals. Take time to think about what it is you need to succeed, but also take time to think about what pitfalls might exist that could facilitate failure. Remember the 5 Ps: Proper Preparation Prevents Poor Performance.

Meal 1 (choose 1 of the following):

- Yogurt parfait made with organic plain Greek yogurt, 2 tablespoons of granola, ⅓ cup of berries and/or sliced banana
- Fruit smoothie (350 calories or less)
- 1½ cups cooked grits (cheese optional)

Meal 2 (choose 1 of the following):

- 1½ cups whole-wheat or whole-grain spaghetti with sun-dried tomatoes (3 to 5 ounces grilled chicken strips or fish optional)

- 1½ cups soup (noncreamy)
- Large green garden salad with 2 tablespoons clean salad dressing (see recipes, pages 223–224)

Meal 3 (choose 1 of the following):

- 6 ounces grilled turkey or skinless chicken with 2 servings of vegetables
- Greens and beans salad made with your greens of choice and black beans, chickpeas, and sunflower seeds
- 6 ounces grilled fish with 2 servings of vegetables

Snacks (choose 3 snacks from below and eat them whenever you want during your feeding window):

- Frozen banana slices (1 whole banana)
- 2 sticks fat-free or low-fat string cheese
- 1 large apple, sliced, sprinkled with cinnamon
- ¼ cup raw mixed nuts
- Watermelon cheese skewers (take 6 toothpicks and on each place 2 cubes watermelon, 1 cube [about the size of one die] feta cheese or your cheese of choice, and 1 slice cucumber)
- 20 raw almonds
- ½ cup organic fat-free or low-fat cottage cheese
- Ten 100% whole-wheat or whole-grain pretzels
- 1 large beefsteak tomato slice and 1 tablespoon crumbled feta cheese
- ½ cup cucumber slices and organic vinaigrette

Work It Out!

> ### *Make an Appointment*
>
> For many of us who lead hectic lives, there are a million excuses for us to not exercise. The best way to stick to a routine is to schedule it just like you would a car appointment or doctor's visit. It's important that you give your workout priority just like you do other things in your daily life. Holding yourself accountable is critical, so finding a workout buddy or a trainer can help you stick to your committment.

Beginner: Workout #1 (page 133)

Intermediate: Workout #1 (page 143)

Advanced: Workout #2 (page 154)

THE MORE YOU KNOW!

ZINC

Helps many enzymes function properly; part of the insulin molecule that helps regulate blood sugars; helps DNA repair as well as immune function, wound healing, and taste perception.

RECOMMENDED DIETARY ALLOWANCE

	Male	Female	Pregnancy	Lactation
19+ years	11 mg	8 mg	11 mg	12 mg

DAY 5

"Perfection is idealistic, but realistic is perfection."

No one and nothing is perfect. Don't hold yourself to an impossible standard only to be disappointed when things don't go as planned. It's all right to have stretch goals, but your feelings must be rooted in reality so that if you don't reach those goals, you don't get discouraged. You are going to make a mistake here and there. You are going to make a bad decision. That is completely normal and expected. The answer is not to throw in the towel and give up, but to persevere and tell yourself that you'll do better next time. There's a reason why the pencil was made with an eraser—everyone makes mistakes, and those mistakes can be corrected.

Meal 1 (choose 1 of the following):

- Large fruit plate of melon, grapes, and banana slices (swap out fruits per your preference) with 6 to 8 ounces 100% plain Greek yogurt, berries, and granola
- Frittata with cheese and your choice of vegetables
- 1½ cups cooked oatmeal, with sliced fruit

Meal 2 (choose 1 of the following):

- 1 cup cooked brown rice or quinoa with 1 cup cooked beans, chickpeas, or lentils (no baked beans with sugar added)
- 1 cup soup (no heavy cream) such as chicken noodle, vegetable, lentil, chickpea, split pea, black bean, tomato basil, minestrone
- 1½ cups whole-wheat or whole-grain spaghetti with your choice of vegetables, seafood, or chicken

Meal 3 (choose 1 of the following):

- 4 servings cooked vegetables—corn, zucchini, black beans, and watercress—with ½ cup cooked quinoa or brown rice
- 6 ounces grilled or baked fish with two servings of vegetables
- 6-ounce turkey burger on 100% whole-wheat or whole-grain bun with cheese, lettuce, and tomato and a green garden salad

Snacks (choose 3 snacks from below and eat them whenever you want during your feeding window):

- 10 walnut halves and 1 sliced kiwi
- 1 cup watermelon and red onion salad
- 1 sliced red pepper with 2 tablespoons hummus
- ½ cup black bean dip and veggie sticks (carrots or celery)
- Small baked sweet potato
- 8 olives stuffed with 1 tablespoon feta or blue cheese
- 8 watermelon and honeydew melon balls
- 16 carrots
- Small green garden salad
- Fresh fruit popsicle (made only from freshly squeezed juice and frozen in cubes)

Work It Out!

Fuel Up

Eating the right foods before a workout can help you perform better and recover faster. Your muscles and soft tissues are about to undergo a lot of physical stress during your exercise session, so it's imperative that you nourish them before the

cont.

challenge. A combination of carbs, protein, and fat is beneficial. Carbs help you maximize your storage of glucose in the form of glycogen. This will be your first fuel source for short- and high-intensity exercise. Fat is your source of fuel for longer and moderate- to low-intensity exercise. Protein will improve and facilitate the building of muscle and help with your recovery.

Beginner: Workout #2 (page 134)

Intermediate: Workout #2 (page 144)

Advanced: Workout #3 (page 155)

THE MORE YOU KNOW!

SELENIUM

Antioxidant that works with vitamin E and fights damaging particles in the body called free radicals. Plays critical roles in reproduction, thyroid hormone metabolism, and DNA synthesis.

RECOMMENDED DIETARY ALLOWANCE

	Male	Female	Pregnancy	Lactation
19–50 years	55 mcg	55 mcg	60 mcg	70 mcg
51+ years	55 mcg	55 mcg		

DAY 6

"A clean mind leads to clear thoughts; a clean body leads to great health and happiness."

Your body is going through many changes as you cleanse your tissues and bloodstream of processed ingredients. Imagine taking a filthy washrag and dropping it in a bucket of hot water and bleach. Enzymatic reactions will take place that will break the bonds of the dirt and their attachment to the fibers of the rag. If it sits there long enough and is subjected to repetitive twisting and turning motions, once you take the rag out of the water, it will look drastically different from what it looked like before it was cleaned. Your internal tissues are that rag, and all the phytonutrients you're eating on this clean program comprise the bleach, and your exercise is the repetitive twisting and turning.

Meal 1 (choose 1 of the following):

- Fruit smoothie (350 calories or less)
- Tropical smoothie bowl (pulse 1½ cups fruit—banana, mango, pineapple—and almond milk until smooth and thick; top with blueberries, fresh kiwi, and peaches)

Meal 2 (choose 1 of the following):

- 1½ cups vegetable, tomato, chicken, lentil, or bean soup with a small green garden salad
- 1 cup whole-wheat or whole-grain pasta with green beans and sun-dried tomatoes (other vegetables and fresh tomatoes can be substituted)

Meal 3 (choose 1 of the following):

- 6-ounce grilled skinless, boneless chicken breast with ½ cup cooked brown rice and ½ cup cooked black beans
- Large green garden salad with copious amounts of protein (protein options: chicken, seafood, beans, nuts, chickpeas, lentils, quinoa)
- 1½ cups whole-wheat or whole-grain pasta with tomatoes, sliced chicken, and veggies

Snacks (choose 3 snacks from below and eat them whenever you want during your feeding window):

- Loaded pepper slices: 1 cup red bell pepper slices topped with ¼ cup warm black beans and 1 tablespoon guacamole
- 1 cup fresh cherries
- 8 to 10 green olives
- ½ cup fat-free or low-fat cottage cheese
- ¼ cup wasabi peas
- 1 cup mixed fruit salad
- 2 slices grilled pineapple
- ½ cup banana slices and 1 tablespoon organic peanut butter
- 15 to 20 unroasted peanuts
- ⅓ cup mashed avocado and 8 carrot sticks

Work It Out!

Make It Fun

There are enough exercises and workout routines available that you can choose ones that are not only effective, but also fun. When exercise feels onerous or like a chore, you are less

cont.

likely to do it or stick with it. So choose a workout that will challenge you, but that you enjoy doing. Even try incorporating it into a game where you try to improve your time or the number of repetitions you complete. Like anything else in life, the more you enjoy something, the more likely you are to do it again.

Beginner: Rest

Intermediate: Rest

Advanced: Rest

THE MORE YOU KNOW!

MAGNESIUM

Extremely abundant in the body and helps with mineralization of bones and teeth, muscle contraction, nerve conduction, normal heart rhythm, and enzyme function.

RECOMMENDED DIETARY ALLOWANCE

	Male	Female	Pregnancy	Lactation
19–30 years	400 mg	310 mg	350 mg	310 mg
31–50 years	420 mg	320 mg	360 mg	320 mg
51+ years	420 mg	320 mg		

DAY 7

"Life without fun is like a car without an engine."

As you complete the first week of your transformation, it's important to remember that having fun is an integral part of living, even when you're focused on making difficult and substantial changes in your life. It's easy to be so serious about doing the right things and following the plan as meticulously as possible that you ignore the joy and fun of being alive. When you continue to have fun on a plan like this, it makes everything easier and you can maintain a better perspective and more positive attitude about what's to come. Don't take yourself too seriously but be willing to laugh at your mistakes and take it in stride when you don't measure up to hopes or expectations. It's worthy to always try your best, but it's important to remember that no one is perfect.

Meal 1 (choose 1 of the following):

- 1 cup fat-free plain Greek yogurt, ¼ cup muesli, ¼ cup blueberries
- Avocado-egg toast (1 slice 100% whole-wheat or whole-grain bread, ¼ mashed medium avocado, 1 egg cooked in ¼ teaspoon olive oil)

Meal 2 (choose 1 of the following):

- Turkey or chicken sandwich on 100% whole-wheat or whole-grain bread with lettuce, tomato, and cheese and a small green garden salad

- 6-ounce veggie burger on 100% whole-wheat or whole-grain bun with lettuce, tomato, and cheese and a small green garden salad

Meal 3 (choose 1 of the following):

- 4 servings of cooked vegetables (black beans, carrots, cabbage, cauliflower) with 1 cup soup such as lentil, chickpea, or chicken
- Turkey lasagna made with whole-wheat or whole-grain noodles and 2 servings of vegetables
- Grilled chicken with quinoa and steamed asparagus (or another vegetable of choice)

Snacks (choose 3 snacks from below and eat them whenever you want during your feeding window):

- Kale chips (½ cup raw kale, stems removed, baked with 1 teaspoon olive oil at 400°F until crisp)
- 1 cup fresh berries
- 20 raw almonds
- 15 walnuts
- ½ grapefruit
- ½ cup sunflower seeds
- ⅓ cup organic, no-sugar-added trail mix
- 1 cup roasted chickpeas tossed with extra-virgin olive oil
- 1 hard-boiled egg with seasoning
- 8-ounce fresh fruit smoothie

Work It Out!

Form Matters

Sometimes it's not *what* you do that counts, but *how* you do it. Performing an exercise the wrong way leaves you vulnerable to injury, and also means you're not maximizing the benefits you can reap from the workout. Learn the proper techniques and employ them even if it means you can't do as many repetitions of the exercise that you're attempting. Don't waste time trying to impress others with how much you can do when what you're doing is not right anyway.

Beginner: Workout #2 (page 134)

Intermediate: Workout #2 (page 144)

Advanced: Workout #2 (page 154)

THE MORE YOU KNOW!

PHOSPHORUS

Helps maintain bones and teeth and is an important component of our DNA and cell membranes. Buffers acids, which helps the body maintain a normal pH. Temporary storage and transfer of energy derived from metabolic fuels.

RECOMMENDED DIETARY ALLOWANCE

	Male	*Female*
19+ years	700 mg	700 mg

DAY 8

*"Some reflection on what you've accomplished
can inspire you to accomplish even more."*

Welcome to the beginning of Week 2! You have spent a week making better decisions, trying new foods, and exercising more regularly. A lot of changes have occurred in this past week, and you might not even be aware of all of them. Take a few minutes before you start your day and reflect on what you've learned about yourself and take stock of what you've been able to accomplish. Allow this to be a source of motivation as you launch into your second week with even bigger and better things ahead.

Meal 1 (choose 1 of the following):

- 2 cups (or less) cold cereal (no sugar added) with milk
- 2-egg omelet with diced vegetables and 2 slices turkey bacon

Meal 2 (choose 1 of the following):

- 5 ounces grilled chicken breast or fish with 1 serving of greens and 1 serving of beans
- 1½ cups turkey, tomato, lentil, bean, or cucumber soup

Meal 3 (choose 1 of the following):

- 6-ounce turkey burger on 100% whole-wheat or whole-grain bun with tomato, lettuce, and cheese and a baked or mashed sweet potato and cauliflower or green beans
- 1½ cups tomato, bean, chickpea, or lentil soup with a small green garden salad

Snacks (choose 3 snacks from below and eat them whenever you want during your feeding window):

- 1 cup shelled edamame
- 3 ounces fresh cooked turkey breast slices and ½ cup raw veggies; if deli turkey slices, make sure it's nitrites/nitrates-free, no antibiotics, artificial flavors, or preservatives
- ½ cup mushrooms marinated in extra-virgin olive oil, salt, and pepper
- 10 to 12 baked sweet potato fries brushed with extra-virgin olive oil and sea salt
- 1 cup mixed fruit salad
- 1 large apple, sliced, with 1 tablespoon almond butter
- Fresh fruit popsicle (made only from freshly squeezed juice and frozen into cubes)
- 2 slices grilled pineapple
- ½ cup banana slices and 1 tablespoon organic peanut butter
- 15 to 20 unroasted peanuts

Work It Out!

Prime Time

When you work out can be as critical as the workout itself. Don't choose a time when you are low in energy or distracted or rushed. Exercising places demands on your body and mind, so the last thing you want to do is create a more stressful environment by working out at a less optimal time. Sometimes you don't have a choice when you work out, so by all means getting in some exercise even in less-than-ideal circumstances is definitely better than not exercising at all.

Beginner: Workout #2 (page 134)

Intermediate: Workout #2 (page 144)

Advanced: Workout #3 (page 155)

THE MORE YOU KNOW!

CHROMIUM

Its actions in the body aren't completely known or well defined, but it's believed to help insulin move glucose from the blood into the cells. It's also believed to play a role in carbohydrate, fat, and protein metabolism.

ADEQUATE DAILY INTAKE:

	Male	*Female*	*Pregnancy*	*Lactation*
19–50 years	35 mcg	25 mcg	30 mcg	45 mcg
51+ years	30 mcg	20 mcg		

DAY 9

"Your only competition is what you see in the mirror."

Too many people fall into the trap of comparison. A friend or a loved one has lost a certain amount of weight or has been able to achieve a change in their physique, and you ask out loud, Why haven't I been able to do the same thing? The best person to compare yourself to . . . is *you*! All of us lose weight differently, and our bodies don't react the same way to the foods we eat or the exercises we perform. It's a big mistake to hear about what someone else has been able to accomplish on a similar program, then feel discouraged or like a failure that you have not been able to achieve the same results. Try to be the best you and don't worry about what others have done.

Meal 1 (choose 1 of the following):

- 2-egg broccoli and cheese omelet
- 2-egg asparagus-mushroom frittata
- Fruit smoothie (350 calories or less)

Meal 2 (choose 1 of the following):

- Large green garden salad with 3 ounces chicken or fish and 2 tablespoons clean salad dressing (see recipes, pages 223–224)
- 1½ cups whole-wheat or whole-grain pasta in tomato sauce with meat and fish options (chicken, turkey meatballs, salmon)

Meal 3 (choose 1 of the following):

- 6 ounces grilled or baked fish with squash or zucchini slices (3 to 5 ounces sliced chicken or fish optional)
- 4 servings of cooked vegetables (spinach, black-eyed peas, sweet potato, and chickpeas)
- 2 slices whole-wheat or whole-grain pizza and a small green garden salad

Snacks (choose 3 snacks from below and eat them whenever you want during your feeding window):

- 1 hard-boiled egg sprinkled with salt and choice of spices (pepper, paprika, etc.)
- ½ cucumber (8 to 10 slices) and 2 tablespoons hummus
- ½ cup raw or cooked vegetables
- ¼ cup walnuts (or peanuts, cashews, almonds, or pecans)
- ¾ cup steamed edamame (in shell)
- 10 cherry tomatoes sprinkled with salt, pepper, and vinaigrette
- 8 watermelon and honeydew melon balls
- 16 baby carrots
- Small green garden salad

Work It Out!

Lift and Get Lean

Strength training is something that is beneficial to all of us, not just men who like to go to the gym or people training for a physique competition. To reap the benefits of strength training, it doesn't mean you have to lift heavy weights or spend hours in the gym. The American Council on Exercise found in a survey that just 20 minutes a day twice a week will help tone the entire body.

Beginner: Rest

Intermediate: Rest

Advanced: Rest

THE MORE YOU KNOW!

IODINE

Critical component of the thyroid hormones thyroxine (T_4) and triiodothyronine (T_3), which regulate growth, development, protein synthesis, enzyme activity, and metabolism.

RECOMMENDED DIETARY ALLOWANCE

	Male	*Female*	*Pregnancy*	*Lactation*
19+ years	150 mcg	150 mcg	220 mcg	220 mcg

DAY 10

"Life begins at the end of your comfort zone."

Push yourself to go to the next level. Gains and improvements to your body don't just happen naturally; rather you must challenge yourself. It's easy to get into a groove and get comfortable eating the same foods and doing the same workouts. While this familiarity makes you feel good, it can also breed a type of complacency that can hinder your progress. Now it's time to kick it up a notch. Dig in a little deeper. Go an extra five seconds during the active phase of your exercise or add another set of repetitions. On a rest day, do 10 minutes of low-intensity or moderate exercise. Most people don't go anywhere near their boundary, so there's plenty of room left for you to go a little harder without crossing the line.

Meal 1 (choose 1 of the following):

- 1 protein shake (350 calories or less)
- 1 fruit smoothie (350 calories or less)
- 1 grilled cheese sandwich made with 100% whole-wheat or whole-grain bread and organic cheese

Meal 2 (choose 1 of the following):

- Tuna salad sandwich on 100% whole-wheat or whole-grain bread with lettuce with ½ cup raw carrots and hummus
- Chicken sandwich on 100% whole-wheat or whole-grain bread with tomato, lettuce, and clean mayo (page 222) and 1 ounce cheese (optional) with a small green garden salad

Meal 3 (choose 1 of the following):

- 1½ cups whole-wheat or whole-grain spaghetti with squash or zucchini slices (3 to 5 ounces diced chicken or fish optional)
- 6-ounce turkey burger on a 100% whole-wheat or -grain bun with 1 slice organic cheese, tomato, and lettuce with 2 servings of cooked vegetables or a medium green salad
- 2 slices whole-wheat or whole-grain pizza and a small green garden salad

Snacks (choose 3 snacks from below and eat them whenever you want during your feeding window):

- 1 rib celery, chopped, and 2 tablespoons hummus
- 1 apple, sliced, with 1 tablespoon organic peanut butter
- ¾ cup melon cubes
- 40 shelled or unshelled pistachios
- 20 seedless grapes with 10 almonds or cashews
- Kale chips (½ cup raw kale, stems removed, baked with 1 teaspoon olive oil at 400°F until crisp)

Work It Out!

Keep Track

Keeping a journal of your wins and losses, progress and setbacks, can be an important tool as you construct your transformation. It's okay to keep your head down in focus as you go about your work, but every so often you need to look up and take an assessment. Your journal should not only include your goals and progress toward them but keep notes about how you're feeling during certain times and self-observations about how you perform your best and what helps you do it. This journal is your blueprint and record keeper all wrapped in one.

Beginner: Workout #3 (page 135)

Intermediate: Workout #3 (page 145)

Advanced: Workout #3 (page 155)

THE MORE YOU KNOW!

VITAMIN A (RETINOL)

Critical for vision, reproduction, and cellular communication. Helps with bone growth, appetite, and taste. Helps regulate the immune system.

RECOMMENDED DIETARY ALLOWANCE

	Male	*Female*	*Pregnancy*	*Lactation*
19–50 years	900 mcg RAE	700 mcg RAE	770 mcg RAE	1,300 mcg RAE
51+ years	900 mcg RAE	700 mcg RAE		

RAE: Retinol Activity Equivalents, which means the amount of vitamin A available afer the body converts the carotenoids into vitamin A.

DAY 11

"Fear is the catalyst for paralysis."

Be fearless. These words look simple on the page, but they are so big and complicated in real life. So often we let our fear of things known and unknown control how we think and what we do. Life is too short to be distracted by this often-misplaced emotion. Being cautious and contemplative is completely fine, and in many instances very necessary, but fear does something deep inside us that sets off a cascade of thoughts and decisions that can be misguided and misinformed. Fear can become a stubborn hindrance to our progress and difficult to eradicate if we allow it to become entrenched in our psyche. On this journey of transformation, embrace your challenges with a confidence and curious exuberance that will allow you to explore new opportunities, broaden your horizons, and give you a reassurance that you really can do it!

Meal 1 (choose 1 of the following):

- 1½ cups oatmeal with fresh berries or bananas (honey and cinnamon optional)
- 2 scrambled eggs with cheese and veggies and 2 slices turkey bacon

Meal 2 (choose 1 of the following):

- 1½ cups soup (chicken, lentil, black bean, cauliflower, or tomato)
- Turkey sandwich on 100% whole-wheat or whole-grain bread with lettuce, tomato, and cheese and 2 servings of cooked vegetables or a small green garden salad

- Grilled cheese sandwich on 100% whole-wheat or whole-grain bread with a small green garden salad

Meal 3 (choose 1 of the following):

- Large green garden salad with 2 tablespoons clean salad dressing (see recipes, pages 223–224) (3 to 5 ounces sliced chicken breast or fish optional)
- 2 cups soup (chicken, lentil, bean, or butternut squash)

Snacks (choose 3 snacks from below and eat them whenever you want during your feeding window):

- 1 slice 100% whole-wheat or whole-grain pita bread, cut into quarters, with 2 tablespoons hummus
- 10 cherries (fresh or dried, but if dried, then no preservatives or other additives) mixed with a handful of nuts (cashews, almonds, or walnuts)
- ½ cup shelled or unshelled pistachios
- 1 large apple, orange, or banana
- 2 small peaches
- 3 cups air-popped popcorn (light seasoning)
- ⅓ cup egg salad made with clean mayonnaise (see mayonnaise recipe, page 222)
- ⅔ cup cauliflower with 2 tablespoons hummus
- 1 fat-free mozzarella cheese stick and 1 small apple
- 1 sliced tomato with a pinch of pepper and/or salt and extra-virgin olive oil

Work It Out!

> # *Hydrate! Hydrate! Hydrate!*
>
> Many people underestimate the need for hydration during exercise and the positive impact it can have on your workout and avoiding injury. Just because you're not dripping with sweat doesn't mean you're not in need of water and electrolyte replenishment. Over the course of exercising there can be lots of "quiet" water loss—you don't see the loss, but your body feels it. Make sure you liberally drink water, and if you're exercising for an extended period of time, find a beverage that also includes electrolytes to replace what your body is using or losing.

Beginner: Workout #3 (page 135)

Intermediate: Workout #3 (page 145)

Advanced: Workout #4 (page 156)

THE MORE YOU KNOW!

VITAMIN B1 (THIAMINE)

Plays a critical role in energy metabolism, thus it's involved in growth, development, and function of cells. Involved in nerve, muscle, and heart function as well as digestion.

RECOMMENDED DIETARY ALLOWANCE

	Male	*Female*	*Pregnancy*	*Lactation*
19–50 years	1.2 mg	1.1 mg	1.4 mg	1.4 mg
51+ years	1.2 mg	1.1 mg		

DAY 12

"An open mind is a blank canvas for great creations."

Open your mind to new tastes and new possibilities when it comes to eating and exercises. We tend to establish routines, because familiar makes us feel good and comfortable. For these thirty days, boldly try foods and combinations that you've otherwise avoided or never even thought of consuming. Don't be afraid to attempt an exercise that you've deemed too complicated or too challenging for your level of fitness. By all means it's important to be safe, but sometimes pushing yourself or your limits is what makes life full and engaging. Remember, life begins at the end of your comfort zone.

Meal 1 (choose 1 of the following):

- Avocado spread on 2 slices 100% whole-wheat or whole-grain bread with 2 slices turkey bacon
- 2 scrambled eggs (cheese and diced vegetables optional) with 2 slices turkey bacon

Meal 2 (choose 1 of the following):

- 6 ounces grilled or baked halibut (or a fish of your preference)
- Large kale salad with nuts and/or shelled sunflower seeds, tomatoes, and orange slices

Meal 3 (choose 1 of the following):

- 6-ounce veggie burger on 100% whole-wheat or whole-grain bread and 2 servings of cooked vegetables
- 6-ounce grilled chicken breast with brown rice and spinach, cabbage, or cauliflower

Snacks (choose 3 snacks from below and eat them whenever you want during your feeding window):

- 1 rib celery, chopped, and 2 tablespoons hummus
- 1 apple, sliced, with 1 tablespoon organic peanut butter
- ¾ cup melon cubes
- Loaded pepper slices (1 cup red bell pepper slices topped with ¼ cup warm black beans and 1 tablespoon guacamole)
- 1 cup fresh cherries
- 8 to 10 green or black olives
- 1 large apple, sliced, sprinkled with cinnamon
- ¼ cup raw mixed nuts
- Watermelon cheese skewers (take 6 toothpicks and on each place 2 cubes watermelon and 1 cube (about the size of one die) feta cheese or your cheese of choice, and 1 slice cucumber)
- 20 raw almonds

Work It Out!

One Mile

One of the best workouts you can do for improving your stamina, burning fat, and increasing muscle tone is to get on a treadmill and run a mile as fast as you can. That's right, just one mile, flat out. If you are not a runner, don't worry. Walk a mile as fast as you can. When you finish the run, you should be able to taste the lactic acid in the back of your mouth and your heart rate should be jumping into the back of your throat. In less than 10 minutes you would've done the work others need triple the time to achieve.

Beginner: Rest

Intermediate: Rest

Advanced: Workout #4 (page 156)

THE MORE YOU KNOW!

VITAMIN B2 (RIBOFLAVIN)

Important for normal vision and skin health as well as nails and eyesight; helps with breakdown of fat and carbohydrates. An essential component of two major coenzymes involved in energy production, cellular function, growth, and development.

RECOMMENDED DIETARY ALLOWANCE

	Male	Female	Pregnancy	Lactation
19–50 years	1.3 mg	1.1 mg	1.4 mg	1.6 mg
51+ years	1.3 mg	1.1 mg		

Day 13

*"Gratitude is a lens that can make the world around you
and all that's in it appear bigger."*

Gratitude is more than just a simple thank you when someone opens the door or lets you first onto a waiting elevator. Gratitude is actually a process that can resonate deep within your soul and provide a reassuring sense of comfort. Looking at your cup half full rather than half empty is more than just a bandied-about cliché. This perspective has significant implications for how you see the world and how you react to difficult situations. As you work hard to transform, remember that it's not just your body and diet that can benefit from these new changes in your life. Regardless of how old you are, your mind is like a piece of clay that can be constantly molded and stretched and reconfigured, which will only add to the strength of your efforts to change.

Meal 1 (choose 1 of the following):

- 1½ cups oatmeal, cooked with ½ teaspoon honey and fruit and 2 slices turkey bacon (optional) with a piece of fruit
- 1½ cups grits with cheese and 2 slices turkey bacon (optional) with a piece of fruit

Meal 2 (choose 1 of the following):

- Chicken sandwich on 100% whole-wheat or whole-grain bread with lettuce, tomato, and cheese and a small green garden salad
- Turkey sandwich on 100% whole-wheat or whole-grain bread with lettuce, tomato, and cheese and a small green garden salad

- Large green garden salad with 2 tablespoons clean salad dressing (see recipes, pages 223–224) (3 to 5 ounces sliced chicken breast or fish optional)

Meal 3 (choose 1 of the following):

- Spinach or vegetable lasagna made with whole-wheat or whole-grain noodles (piece of lasagna no bigger than 5 by 4 inches, and 2 inches thick)
- 6 ounces turkey with 2 servings of vegetables

Snacks (choose 3 snacks from below and eat them whenever you want during your feeding window):

- 10 walnut halves and 1 sliced kiwi
- 1 cup watermelon and red onion salad
- 1 sliced red pepper with 2 tablespoons hummus
- 2 dates stuffed with almonds (take out the pits and replace with 2 almonds)
- 3 tomato slices and fresh basil drizzled with extra-virgin olive oil
- 8 baby carrots with 2 tablespoons hummus
- 1 slice 100% whole-wheat or whole-grain pita bread, cut into quarters with 2 tablespoons hummus
- 1 cup fresh berries
- 20 raw almonds
- 15 walnuts

Work It Out!

Bookend Your Workout

College and professional athletes who are trying to maximize results from a training program will do something called

cont.

bookend workouts. What this means is that they'll do a workout early in the day, then, later in the afternoon or evening, they'll do another workout that is less intense, but still provides some challenge. Choose one or two days a week where you try this. Not only will this help results come faster, but it will increase the length of time your body spends in fat-burning, calorie-consuming mode throughout the day. It's probably best not to do bookend workouts on consecutive days unless you are working completely different body parts.

Beginner: Workout #4 (page 136)

Intermediate: Workout #4 (page 146)

Advanced: Rest

THE MORE YOU KNOW!

VITAMIN B3 (NIACIN)

Important for digestive system, nervous system, and skin health. Involved in enzymatic reactions that produce energy through the process of degrading carbohydrates, fats, proteins, and alcohol.

RECOMMENDED DIETARY ALLOWANCE

	Male	Female	Pregnancy	Lactation
19–50 years	16 mg	14 mg	18 mg	17 mg
51+	16 mg	14 mg		

DAY 14

*"Understanding lessons of the past can be a
great education for the future."*

Congratulations on reaching the end of your second week.
This is a great time to take a few minutes and review some of the
goals that you set before starting this journey. This is a time to step
back and take a landscape view of how far you've come and what's
ahead of you, to figure out what is working for you and what's not.
If you need to make some tweaks and modifications in what you're
doing based on what you've learned the last couple of weeks, go
ahead and do it. You now have two weeks of hard-earned experience to draw from, so make good use of it as you prepare to tackle
the second half of this journey.

Meal 1 (choose 1 of the following):

- Fruit smoothie (350 calories or less)
- Protein shake (350 calories or less)

Meal 2 (choose 1 of the following):

- Spinach lasagna made with whole-wheat or whole-grain
  noodles (piece of lasagna no bigger than 5 by 4 inches,
  and 2 inches thick)
- 1½ cups soup (carrot, cucumber, chicken, or turkey) with
  a small green garden salad

Meal 3 (choose 1 of the following):

- 6-ounce grilled or baked chicken breast with 2 servings
  of vegetables

- 6-ounce grilled or baked fish with 2 servings of vegetables
- 4 servings of cooked vegetables of your choice

Snacks (choose 3 snacks from below and eat them whenever you want during your feeding window):

- 10 walnut halves and 1 sliced kiwi
- 1 cup watermelon and red onion salad
- 1 sliced red pepper with 2 tablespoons hummus
- ½ cup black bean dip and 8 veggie sticks (carrots or celery)
- Small baked sweet potato
- 1 cup mixed fruit salad
- 1 large apple, sliced, with 1 tablespoon almond butter
- 3 ounces fresh cooked turkey breast slices and raw veggies or, if deli turkey slices, make sure it's nitrites/nitrates-free, no antibiotics, no artificial flavors, no preservatives
- 1 cup fresh berries
- 20 raw almonds

Work It Out!

Warm Up and Cool Down

Don't make the mistake of jumping right into an exercise. This causes many avoidable injuries. Try some stretching, making sure you go through the motions of the exercise you're about to do, focusing on those muscles you will be using. When you're done, it's also important to go through a cool-down. Take a few minutes to stretch the muscles and joints that you just worked.

Beginner: Workout #4 (page 136)

Intermediate: Workout #4 (page 146)

Advanced: Workout #4 (page 156)

THE MORE YOU KNOW!

VITAMIN B5 (PANTOTHENIC ACID)

Plays a role in the breakdown of fats and carbohydrates for energy. Important for manufacture of red blood cells as well as sex and stress-related hormones produced in adrenal glands.

RECOMMENDED DIETARY ALLOWANCE

	Male	*Female*	*Pregnancy*	*Lactation*
19+ years	5 mg	5 mg	6 mg	7 mg

DAY 15

"One of the most important things about reaching a goal is actually taking the time to celebrate what you've worked so hard to accomplish."

Congrats on reaching the midway point of your journey! This is a really big accomplishment and you should take a moment to applaud your efforts. Think back to when you were about to start your first day and reflect on the thoughts that were going through your mind and the concerns you had about undergoing this transformation. Now take a look at yourself and how far you've come. Let this be a confirmation that you can accomplish whatever you truly set your mind to do, and motivation to keep working at the program, getting better at what you're doing and being more determined to reach other goals. Reward yourself for a job well done and be encouraged that there are more sunrises ahead.

Meal 1 (choose 1 of the following):

- Yogurt parfait with a piece of fruit
- 2-egg omelet with cheese and vegetables of choice, with a piece of fruit

Meal 2 (choose 1 of the following):

- Baja salad (mixture of 4-ounce grilled skinless chicken breast, chopped; 1 medium tomato, diced; ¼ cup cooked black beans; ½ avocado, diced; 1 tablespoon chopped red onion; 1 teaspoon cilantro leaves; 1 tablespoon extra-virgin olive oil; juice of 1 lime)
- Large green garden salad with chickpeas, olives, and tomatoes

Meal 3 (choose 1 of the following):

- 6-ounce grilled skinless, boneless chicken breast or salmon with ½ cup cooked brown rice and ½ cup cooked black beans
- 1½ cup whole-wheat or whole-grain spaghetti with squash or zucchini slices (3 to 5 ounces diced chicken or fish optional)
- 4 servings of vegetables of your choice

Snacks (choose 3 snacks from below and eat them whenever you want during your feeding window):

- Frozen banana slices (1 whole banana)
- 2 sticks fat-free or low-fat string cheese
- 1 large apple, sliced, sprinkled with cinnamon
- ¼ cup raw mixed nuts or 15 cashews
- Watermelon cheese skewers (take 6 toothpicks and on each place 2 cubes watermelon and 1 cube [about the size of one die] feta cheese or your cheese of choice, and 1 slice cucumber)
- 20 raw almonds
- one 8-ounce fresh smoothie
- ½ cup black bean dip and 8 veggie sticks (carrots or celery)

Work It Out!

Try a Pro

While you might not have the disposable income to have training sessions on a continual basis, there is definitely a benefit to having at least a couple of sessions. Trainers can not only teach you proper form so that you are doing the exercises safely

cont.

and effectively, but they can help build and customize workouts that best fit your body, goals, and needs. Just a couple of sessions could yield dramatic differences in what you achieve.

Beginner: Rest

Intermediate: Rest

Advanced: Rest

VITAMIN B5 (PANTOTHENIC ACID)

One fast way to cut calories and lose weight is to reduce the amount of added sugars you consume. According to the National Institutes of Health, the average American consumes 152 pounds of sugar in just one year, which means 3 pounds (or 6 cups) consumed in one week. It's easy to calculate how many teaspoons of sugar are contained in whatever you eat or drink. Every teaspoon of sugar contains 4 grams. Look at the nutrition label and find the number of grams of sugar, then divide that number by 4. The resulting number is how many teaspoons of sugar are in each serving of that product. For example, if a can of soda contains 39 grams of sugar in one 12 oz bottle, then there are 9.7 teaspoons of sugar in just that one bottle. Do the simple math before you eat and drink and you could save mightily on your calorie consumption!

DAY 16

*"Decisions don't have an expiration date;
their impact can last forever."*

Life is like a revolving carousel of decisions. Every day we make thousands of decisions, some trivial, others that can mean the difference between life and death. Many of these decisions are simple reflexes. You're crossing the street and a car turns the corner and starts barreling in your direction. Without even thinking, you immediately run to the other side of the street to get out of the way. Then there are those decisions to which you give conscious thought, such as sitting in a restaurant looking at a menu deciding what to eat. Lots of thoughts inform your ultimate decision, and you take your time to wrestle with these thoughts until comfortable with your order. Sometimes it's important to remember the long-term implications of your decisions, even when immediate gratification is right within your grasp. Junk food, whether it's a rich chocolate bar or greasy fast food, provides immediate satisfaction to our senses of taste, touch, and smell. But that immediate gratification could also lead to long-term consequences that come at a steep price, one you typically would not want to pay for one slice of chocolate cake. Surely, life is meant to be fun, but when deciding what kind of fun you want to have, sometimes it's best to take the long view instead of what's right in front of you.

Meal 1 (choose 1 of the following):

- 1½ cups cooked oatmeal with fresh berries or banana (honey and cinnamon optional)

- 1 scrambled egg with cheese and veggies and 2 slices turkey bacon

Meal 2 (choose 1 of the following):

- 1½ cups turkey or chicken chili with a small green garden salad
- Turkey sandwich on 100% whole-wheat or whole-grain bread with lettuce, tomato, and cheese and a small green garden salad

Meal 3 (choose 1 of the following):

- 6-ounce veggie burger on 100% whole-wheat or whole-grain bread and 2 servings of cooked vegetables
- 1½ cups whole-wheat or whole-grain spaghetti with squash or zucchini slices (3 to 5 ounces diced chicken or fish optional)
- 6-ounce turkey burger with 1 slice organic cheese, lettuce, and tomato with 2 servings of cooked vegetables or a medium green garden salad

Snacks (choose 3 snacks from below and eat them whenever you want during your feeding window):

- 1 large apple, orange, or banana
- 2 small peaches
- 3 cups plain air-popped popcorn (light seasoning)
- 1 cup fresh berries
- 20 raw almonds
- 15 walnuts
- ½ grapefruit
- 1 nonfat mozzarella cheese stick with 1 small apple
- Sliced tomatoes with a pinch of pepper and/or salt and olive oil
- Ten 100% whole-wheat or whole-grain pretzels

Work It Out!

Define Your Goals

It's important when following an exercise regimen to always have a sense of where you are. This is not about competing with a friend or colleague or someone else at the gym; rather this is about you knowing your progress and setting goals to keep you motivated to go further and challenge yourself. Keep a list in your phone or on your fridge and check it out once a day.

Beginner: Workout #4 (page 136)

Intermediate: Workout #4 (page 146)

Advanced: Workout #5 (page 157)

THE MORE YOU KNOW!

COMMON DIETARY SOURCES OF FIBER

Apples	Leafy green vegetables
Barley	Legumes (beans)
Beans	Lentils
Blueberries	Nuts and seeds
Brown rice	Oatmeal, oat bran
Bulgur	Pears
Carrots	Strawberries
Celery	Tomatoes
Couscous	Wheat bran
Cucumbers	Whole-wheat or whole-grain
Dried peas	breakfast cereals and breads

DAY 17

"Living in your past could mean the end of your living."

It's our natural instinct to dwell on things that have happened in the past. Whether it's a mistake on a test, an argument with a loved one, or a decision that has brought painful consequences, we tend to spend an inordinate amount of time thinking about all that has gone wrong. The simple truth is that the past is the past, and regardless of how hard you try to mentally rearrange things, it can't be undone. But what you do have control over is what is in your future. There's certainly nothing wrong with an occasional look in your rearview mirror, as it can give you context for what you need to do or things you need to avoid going forward. But this look must be for the purpose of informing rather than the purpose of shaming yourself for past failings. Too often we allow our minds to be so cluttered with what happened years, months, or weeks ago that there's little if any room to focus on the wide-open road waiting ahead of us. There is a natural excitement that comes with exploring the unknown and untraveled and unexpected. Use your energy to chart a new course, learn new things, and establish a new trajectory that will bring you happiness and hope for great things yet to come.

Meal 1 (choose 1 of the following):

- 2 cups (or less) cold cereal (no sugar added) with milk
- 2-egg omelet with diced vegetables and 2 slices turkey bacon

Meal 2 (choose 1 of the following):

- 1½ cups soup (vegetable, tomato, chicken, lentil, or bean) with a small green garden salad
- 5 ounces grilled chicken breast or fish with 1 serving of greens and 1 serving of beans

Meal 3 (choose 1 of the following):

- 1½ cups whole-wheat or whole-grain spaghetti with squash or zucchini slices (3 to 5 ounces diced chicken or fish optional)
- 4 servings of cooked vegetables (spinach, black-eyed peas, sweet potato, and chickpeas)
- 2 slices whole-wheat or whole-grain pizza and a small green garden salad

Snacks (choose 3 snacks from below and eat them whenever you want during your feeding window):

- 8 baby carrots with 2 tablespoons hummus
- 1 slice whole-wheat or whole-grain pita bread, cut into quarters, with 2 tablespoons hummus
- 10 cherries mixed with a handful of nuts (cashews, almonds, or walnuts)
- ½ cup black bean dip and 8 veggie sticks (carrots or celery)
- Small baked sweet potato
- 8 olives stuffed with 1 tablespoon feta or blue cheese
- Loaded pepper slices (1 cup red bell pepper slices topped with ¼ cup warm black beans and 1 tablespoon guacamole)
- 1 cup fresh cherries
- 8 to 10 green or black olives

Work It Out!

> ### *Benefits of Resistance Training*
>
> Improves strength and balance
>
> Improves protection against physical injury
>
> Improves diabetes management
>
> Prevents osteoporosis (bone thinning)
>
> Helps prevent/manage cardiovascular disease such as heart attacks, stroke, artery disease, and heart failure
>
> Improves functioning and mobility in arthritis sufferers

Beginner: Workout #5 (page 137)

Intermediate: Workout #5 (page 147)

Advanced: Workout #5 (page 157)

THE MORE YOU KNOW!

SUBSTITUTIONS MATTER

Swap Out	Try	Calories Saved (1 serving)
Mayonnaise (1 teaspoon)	Mustard	54
Buttered popcorn (1 cup)	Air-popped popcorn	108
Mashed potatoes (1 cup)	Mashed cauliflower	116
Ice cream (½ cup)	Nonfat frozen yogurt	153
Ground beef (4 ounces)	Ground turkey	132

DAY 18

"Don't let failure be a dead end, try another road."

There is often not a lot that separates someone who succeeds from someone who fails. It's easy to think the answer is that someone is smarter or more talented or luckier. But the simple truth is that the difference between those who win and those who lose is old-fashioned tenacity, an extreme persistence in adhering to or doing something. This is not something we're born with; rather it's a characteristic we all have the ability to develop. Think about the countless inspirational stories of people who have repeatedly failed at something but continued to try it again until they found success. There's the bestselling author whose manuscript got rejected fifty times before finding that one editor who believed in it, published it, and watched the book soar to the bestseller list. There's the actress who went to a hundred casting calls without success before finally landing that one role that eventually won her an Emmy. It's definitely not easy to fail then summon the energy and courage to try again. But take a look at the alternative and the answer is staring right back at you. There are never any guarantees when you try, but there is a guarantee that not trying means you will never succeed.

Meal 1 (choose 1 of the following):

- Turkey bacon, egg, and cheese sandwich on 100% whole-wheat or whole-grain bread with a side of fruit
- 1½ cups cooked oatmeal with a side of fruit (honey and cinnamon allowed)

- 2 scrambled eggs with cheese and/or veggies and 1 slice 100% whole-wheat or whole-grain toast

Meal 2 (choose 1 of the following):

- 1½ cups whole-wheat or whole-grain spaghetti with sun-dried tomatoes (3 to 5 ounces grilled chicken strips or fish optional)
- 1½ cups soup (noncreamy)
- Large green garden salad with 2 tablespoons clean salad dressing (see recipes, pages 223–224)

Meal 3 (choose 1 of the following):

- 1½ cups soup (turkey, tomato, lentil, bean, or cucumber)
- 6 ounces grilled or baked fish with squash or zucchini slices (3 to 5 ounces sliced chicken or fish optional)
- 2 slices whole-wheat or -grain pizza, small garden salad

Snacks (choose 3 snacks from below and eat them whenever you want during your feeding window):

- 1 cup mixed fruit salad
- ⅔ cup raw veggies with guacamole
- 15 frozen grapes
- Kale chips (½ cup raw kale, stems removed, baked with 1 teaspoon olive oil at 400°F until crisp)
- 1 cup fresh berries
- 20 raw almonds
- 15 walnuts
- ½ grapefruit
- ½ cup shelled or unshelled sunflower seeds
- 3 cups air-popped popcorn (light seasoning)

Work It Out!

> ## *Calorie Burners*
>
> Look at these exercises and the average amount of calories burned in 1 hour of that activity.
>
> | | |
> |---|---|
> | Running 8 mph | 986 |
> | Rollerblading | 913 |
> | Tae kwon do | 730 |
> | Jumping rope | 730 |
> | Tennis, singles | 584 |
> | Jogging 5 mph | 584 |
> | Swimming laps | 511 |
> | Hiking | 438 |
> | Water aerobics | 292 |

Beginner: Rest

Intermediate: Rest

Advanced: Rest

THE MORE YOU KNOW!

LEGUMES

This is a class of vegetables that includes beans, peas, and lentils. Legumes are extremely versatile in how they can be prepared and are some of the most nutritious foods you can eat. They are typically low in fat, contain no cholesterol, and provide large quantities of folate, potassium, iron, and magnesium. If you're seeking more protein in your diet, legumes are a great source and a good substitute for red meat.

Day 19

"The most potent antidote to doubt is doing."

Too often we set goals in life that fall within our comfort zone, but don't demand that we stretch our mind or abilities. It's important to set goals that can be reached, but it's equally important to set goals that require us to reach beyond what we already know to be doable. Today think of an aspect of your life that you want to improve. It could be improving your punctuality, losing weight, or becoming better organized. Now think about an ultimate goal, one that you can't accomplish in just a week or two, but something that is going to require you to be dedicated and focused to make small improvements for at least a month. You might want to get to work on time for 4 weeks straight without a day being late. You could set a goal of losing 10 pounds in a month with the ultimate goal of losing 30 pounds in three months. Whatever goal you set, make sure that it's going to require significant enough effort such that if you don't focus and give it your best it simply will not be attainable. You don't want to be unrealistic, such as run a marathon in two months when you have never run a marathon before. But within reason, the more you demand of yourself the higher the level of personal accomplishment when you reach your goal. Sometimes it's important to show yourself you can do things, especially when you had doubts about whether it was possible.

Meal 1 (choose 1 of the following):

- Avocado spread on 2 slices 100% whole-wheat or whole-grain bread with 2 slices turkey bacon

- 2 scrambled eggs (cheese and diced vegetables optional) with 2 slices turkey bacon

Meal 2 (choose 1 of the following):

- Turkey sandwich on 100% whole-grain bread with 5 ounces turkey, with the option of 1 ounce cheese, lettuce, tomato, and organic mustard or clean mayonnaise (see recipe, page 222) and a side serving of raw or cooked vegetables
- Large green garden salad with 2 tablespoons clean salad dressing (see recipes, pages 223–224) (3 to 5 ounces sliced chicken breast or fish optional)

Meal 3 (choose 1 of the following):

- 1 cup whole-wheat or whole-grain pasta with cooked vegetables and 3 to 5 ounces diced chicken
- 5-ounce turkey burger on 100% whole-wheat or whole-grain bun with lettuce, tomato, and onion with a medium green garden salad
- 5-ounce chicken burger on 100% whole-wheat or whole-grain bun with lettuce, tomato, and onion with a medium green garden salad

Snacks (choose 3 snacks from below and eat them whenever you want during your feeding window):

- ¼ cup mushrooms marinated in extra-virgin olive oil, salt, and pepper
- 4 clean turkey meatballs (1-inch diameter)
- ¼ cup baked apple chips
- 1 fat-free mozzarella cheese stick with 1 small apple
- 1 sliced tomato with a pinch of pepper and/or salt and olive oil

- Ten 100% whole-wheat or whole-grain pretzels
- 1 large beefsteak tomato slice and 1 tablespoon feta cheese
- 1 cup cooked chickpeas tossed with extra-virgin olive oil and roasted
- 1 hard-boiled egg with seasoning
- 8-ounce fresh fruit smoothie

Dumbbells Are Smart

Adding dumbbells to your exercise routine is a great way to increase the dimensionality to your workout. Building lean muscle mass can be done by people of all sizes and ages. This lean muscle will increase your metabolism, as it requires more energy to feed and sustain muscle. Light dumbbells, where you can do 12 to 15 repetitions of an exercise, are enough to build that nice lean musculature that will make you not only feel better but look better too.

Work It Out!

Beginner: Workout #5 (page 137)

Intermediate: Workout #5 (page 147)

Advanced: Workout #5 (page 157)

THE MORE YOU KNOW!

WHOLE-GRAIN BREAKDOWN

There are three parts to a whole grain:

Bran (outer layer): contains fiber (insoluble), B vitamins, trace minerals, phytochemicals, protein

Endosperm (inner): contains carbohydrate, protein, fiber (soluble)

Germ (embryo): contains vitamin E and healthy fats, B vitamins, protein

DAY 20

"When you're winning, fight like you're losing."

One of the biggest trap holes of success is complacency. When everything seems to be going your way and you're hitting your benchmarks, it's easy to sit back and coast because you start focusing more on the joys and benefits of success rather than the work and energy that it has taken to produce it. It's a common phenomenon in sports. A team will be winning the game by a large margin and then start to become too comfortable. They start smiling and joking on the sidelines, stop paying attention to the details of execution, and start believing that their opponent is too inferior to stage a comeback charge. As the game goes on, the opponents gradually stop making the mistakes they've been making, they refocus their efforts, and a little bit of luck they hadn't been having suddenly starts falling their way. The team that was winning is suddenly caught off guard and can't get back on track fast enough to slow their opponents' momentum that is now overtaking them. When you are winning, it's okay to have some enjoyment, but you must also work even harder and smarter to execute your strategy better to keep winning. Whether you're a tennis player in a grueling five-set match, a marathon runner, or someone trying to lose weight, you must focus and fight the entire distance until the competition is over.

Meal 1 (choose 1 of the following):

- Large fruit plate of melon, grapes, and banana slices (swap out fruits per your preference) with 6 to 8 ounces 100% plain Greek yogurt, berries, and granola
- Frittata with cheese and your choice of vegetables
- 1½ cups cooked oatmeal, with sliced fruit

Meal 2 (choose 1 of the following):

- 6-ounce beef burger on 100% whole-wheat or whole-grain bun with cheese, lettuce, and tomato and a green garden salad
- 6-ounce turkey burger on 100% whole-wheat or whole-grain bun with cheese, lettuce, and tomato and a green garden salad
- Large green garden salad (3 to 5 ounces chicken or fish optional)

Meal 3 (choose 1 of the following):

- Large green garden salad with copious amounts of protein (chicken, seafood, beans, nuts, chickpeas, lentils, quinoa)
- 1½ cups whole-wheat or whole-grain pasta with tomatoes, sliced chicken, and veggies
- 6-ounce turkey burger on 100% whole-wheat or whole-grain bun with cheese, lettuce, and tomato and a green garden salad

Snacks (choose 3 snacks from below and eat them whenever you want during your feeding window):

- Kale chips (½ cup raw kale, stems removed, baked with 1 teaspoon olive oil at 400°F until crisp)
- 1 cup fresh berries
- 20 raw almonds
- 15 walnuts

- ½ grapefruit
- ½ cup shelled or unshelled sunflower seeds
- Ten 100% whole-wheat or whole-grain pretzels
- ½ cup raw veggies and 2 tablespoons guacamole
- 2 sticks low-fat string cheese
- 8–10 green olives

Work It Out!

> ### *Clean It Out*
>
> One of the best ways to find success in your exercise program is to make sure you're not being thrown off by environmental distractions. Clean out your life both literally and figuratively. Clean your cabinets of bad, tempting food. Clean your relationships of people who are naysayers or conduits of temptation.

Beginner: Workout #5 (page 137)

Intermediate: Workout #5 (page 147)

Advanced: Workout #6 (page 158)

THE MORE YOU KNOW!

NAMES FOR ADDED SUGARS

Anhydrous dextrose	Inversol
Brown sugar	Isomalt
Cane sugar	Lactose
Corn sweetener	Malted barley
Corn syrup	Maltose

cont.

Dextrose	Malt syrup
Evaporated cane sugar	Molasses
Fructose	Rice sugar, rice malt
Fruit juice blend	Raw sugar
Fruit juice concentrates	Sorghum
Galactose	Sucanet
Glucose	Sucrose
High-fructose corn syrup	Sugar
Honey	Syrup

DAY 21

"Airplanes are made to be flown, pianos are made to be played, bodies are made to move."

Movement is your best friend, even beyond your scheduled exercise. Try walking during lunch or at home around the neighborhood or even in the local mall when the weather outside isn't cooperating. The more your body moves and muscles contract and heart rate picks up, the better your physiologic state. Little things can make a difference—taking a few flights of steps when possible instead of the elevator, walking a distance you otherwise would've covered riding a bus, taking a ten-minute walk after dinner. Regardless of how you choose to do it, keep yourself moving all day and you will begin to see the results not only in your increased stamina, but in the mirror as well.

Meal 1 (choose 1 of the following):

- Fruit smoothie (350 calories or less)
- Protein shake (350 calories or less)
- 1½ cups cooked grits with 1 ounce cheese and 2 slices turkey bacon (optional) and 1 piece of fruit

Meal 2 (choose 1 of the following):

- 1½ cups whole-wheat or whole-grain spaghetti with sun-dried tomatoes (3 to 5 ounces grilled chicken strips or fish optional)
- 1½ cups soup (noncreamy)
- Large green garden salad with 2 tablespoons clean salad dressing (see recipes, pages 223–224)

Meal 3 (choose 1 of the following):

- Spinach lasagna made with whole-wheat or whole-grain noodles (no bigger than 5 by 4 inches, and 2 inches thick)
- 6 ounces turkey with 2 servings of vegetables
- 6-ounce veggie burger on 100% whole-wheat or whole-grain bread with 2 servings of cooked vegetables

Snacks (choose 3 snacks from below and eat them whenever you want during your feeding window):

- ¼ cup mushrooms marinated in extra-virgin olive oil, salt, and pepper
- 4 clean turkey meatballs (1-inch diameter)
- ¼ cup baked apple chips
- 1 large beefsteak tomato slice and 1 tablespoon feta cheese
- ½ cup cucumber slices and organic vinaigrette dressing
- 8 watermelon and honeydew melon balls
- 3 cups air-popped popcorn (light seasoning)
- 1 cup mixed fruit salad
- ⅔ cup raw veggies with 2 tablespoons guacamole
- 20 raw almonds

Work It Out!

Mix It Up

Change it up and introduce a new challenge to your body. Alter the actual exercise or change the pattern and sequence of the workout. If you've been working out in a gym, try doing what you can outside. The more you mix up your program and your workout environment, the better you will work a broader range

cont.

of muscles in a different way to improve strength and toning. Try something you haven't done before, even if it means a more complicated exercise that you weren't able to do when you first started, but probably can do now. Variation is a catalyst for improvements.

Beginner: Workout #5 (page 137)

Intermediate: Workout #5 (page 147)

Advanced: Workout #5 (page 157)

THE MORE YOU KNOW!

THE BIG 4

Fat	9 calories per gram
Alcohol	7 calories per gram
Carbohydrates	4 calories per gram
Protein	4 calories per gram

DAY 22

"One way to guarantee you won't win is by standing on the sidelines."

When you look at successful people from across the spectrum, one thing you will almost always read in their story is that they believed in themselves, their vision, or their chances of accomplishing a goal. While hope is always essential in the formula of optimism, belief must be more than that. Deep within your being you must truly believe that you can accomplish the dream or goal that is before you. Without this visceral belief, you are vulnerable to the many discouragements and distractions that are constantly trying to tell you that you can't accomplish your goals or succeed. An environment of negativity seems to be easier to create for some than an environment of positivity. It seems like others revel in the opportunity to tell you that you won't or can't succeed or that what you want is unrealistic and irrational. Unfortunately, you must come to expect a certain degree of doubt and nonsupport from others. But those who have succeeded against the odds will quickly tell you that despite the storm that surrounded them, they always believed deep down that they could win. Always believe in yourself first, and that belief will shield you, console you, and nourish your passion so that success is not just a hope but a reality. People who believe in themselves don't stand around and talk about winning. They get in the game.

Meal 1 (choose 1 of the following):

- Large fruit plate of melon, grapes, and banana slices (swap out fruits per your preference) with 6 to 8 ounces 100% plain Greek yogurt, berries, and granola
- Frittata with cheese and your choice of vegetables
- 1½ cups cooked oatmeal, with sliced fruit

Meal 2 (choose 1 of the following):

- Turkey sandwich on 100% whole-wheat or whole-grain bread with 3 to 5 ounces turkey, with 1 ounce cheese (optional), tomato, lettuce, and organic mustard or clean mayonnaise (see recipe, page 222) and a side serving of raw or cooked vegetables
- Large green garden salad with 2 tablespoons clean salad dressing (see recipes, pages 223–224) (3 to 5 ounces sliced chicken breast or fish optional)

Meal 3 (choose 1 of the following):

- 5-ounce veggie burger on 100% whole-wheat or whole-grain bun with lettuce, tomato, and onion with a medium green garden salad
- 5-ounce turkey burger on 100% whole-wheat or whole-grain bun with lettuce, tomato, and onion with a medium green garden salad
- 5-ounce chicken burger on 100% whole-wheat or whole-grain bun with lettuce, tomato, and onion with a medium green garden salad

Snacks (choose 3 snacks from below and eat them whenever you want during your feeding window):

- ¾ cup melon cubes
- 40 shelled or unshelled pistachios

- 20 seedless grapes with 10 almonds or cashews
- Kale chips (½ cup raw kale, stems removed, baked with 1 teaspoon olive oil at 400°F until crisp)
- 1 hard-boiled egg sprinkled with salt and choice of spices (pepper, paprika, etc.)
- ½ cucumber (8 to 10 slices) and 2 tablespoons hummus
- ½ cup raw or cooked vegetables
- ¼ cup walnuts (or peanuts, cashews, almonds, or pecans)
- ¾ cup steamed edamame (in shell)
- 10 cherry tomatoes sprinkled with salt, pepper, and vinaigrette

Work It Out!

Recovery Meal

What you eat after a workout is just as important as what you eat before exercising. Your muscles need the best nourishment to recover and grow, and this means supplying them with carbohydrates and protein. The carbs will replace the glycogen stores that have been depleted with exercise, and the protein will help with muscle growth. Try eating your meal within 60 minutes of finishing your workout.

Beginner: Rest

Intermediate: Rest

Advanced: Rest

THE MORE YOU KNOW!

ADDING GOOD CARBS TO YOUR DIET

Instead of snacking on chips and pretzels, just try some crunchy veggies like carrots, celery, or sliced cucumbers. Dip them in organic peanut butter to add some protein. Also, make it a goal to eat 2 servings of fruit each day. Consume at least one piece in the morning, and for lunch or dinner slice an apple, pear, orange, or other fruit over your salad. Add ½ cup berries to your low-fat yogurt.

DAY 23

*"Food is sustenance and fuel to be used wisely
and not taken for granted or abused."*

What is your relationship to food? Do you eat because
you're depressed and need comfort? When you're stressed, do you
reach for that big bag of potato chips? Are you a social eater, someone who attends a lot of functions where there's always food
around? Are you someone who is lonely and finds food to be a
quiet, reliable companion? When it comes to making better food
choices and losing weight, defining and understanding your relationship to food is extremely important. Eating should be with
purpose, and not as a secondary thing to do while you're doing
something else and want to keep busy. This type of mindless
eating—eating just because the food is there—can be a habit that
you can identify and, with a little effort, break for good. To become a more intentional eater, think about when you eat and why
you eat. Think about your hunger level when you eat and avoid
eating when your body really isn't asking to be fed. There's an old
saying that you should "eat with your stomach and not your eyes."
That is not only true but can prevent you from overindulging at
the most inopportune times. Food is sustenance and fun. Remaining intentional as you select what you eat and how much you eat
will help you make better choices when it comes to fueling your
body.

Meal 1 (choose 1 of the following):

- Turkey bacon, egg, and cheese sandwich on 100% whole-wheat or whole-grain bread with a side of fruit (1 cup diced fruit or 1 piece of fruit)
- 1½ cups cooked oatmeal, with a side of fruit (honey and cinnamon allowed)
- 2 scrambled eggs with cheese and/or veggies and a slice of 100% whole-wheat or whole-grain toast

Meal 2 (choose 1 of the following):

- Chicken or turkey sandwich on 100% whole-wheat or whole-grain bread with lettuce, tomato, cheese, and clean mayo (see recipe, page 222) or mustard, with 1 serving of vegetables or a small green garden salad
- Large green garden salad (3 to 5 ounces chicken or fish optional)

Meal 3 (choose 1 of the following):

- 6 ounces grilled turkey or skinless chicken with 2 servings of vegetables
- Greens and beans salad made with your greens of choice and black beans, chickpeas, and sunflower seeds
- 6 ounces grilled fish of your choice with 2 servings of vegetables

Snacks (choose 3 snacks from below and eat them whenever you want during your feeding window):

- 1 rib celery, chopped, and 2 tablespoons hummus
- 1 apple, sliced, with 1 tablespoon organic peanut butter
- ¾ cup melon cubes
- 40 shelled or unshelled pistachios

- 20 seedless grapes with 10 almonds or cashews
- Loaded pepper slices (1 cup red bell pepper slices topped with ¼ cup warm black beans and 1 tablespoon guacamole)
- 1 cup fresh cherries
- 8 to 10 green or black olives
- ½ cup organic fat-free or low-fat cottage cheese
- ¼ cup wasabi peas

Work It Out!

Gear Up

Don't underestimate the importance of what you wear when working out. Too many people wear the wrong sneakers or clothes that are not conducive to proper movement during exercise. You need footwear that is going to be supportive, but light and flexible at the same time to give you maximal range of motion. You need clothes that are loose enough that they won't restrict your movement, made of breathable material that reduces the amount of sweating or that dries quickly. A wearable device that can keep track of your steps and even calories burned can provide good information to harness for a more productive workout session.

Beginner: Workout #3 (page 135)

Intermediate: Workout #4 (page 146)

Advanced: Workout #5 (page 157)

THE MORE YOU KNOW!

VISUAL MEASUREMENTS

Here are some visual cues for appropriate portion sizes:

Food Item	Physical Equivalent
1 cup cereal flakes	Baseball
½ cup cooked rice	Lightbulb
1 baked sweet potato	Computer mouse
6 ounces lean meat	2 decks of cards

Day 24

"Life is bigger than everything, for without life there is nothing."

Focus on a hobby, anything other than food or exercise. Sometimes we get so determined to succeed on this transformation journey that we forget there's more to life than looking at food labels, watching portion sizes, and trying to complete yet another exercise session. It's important to keep everything in perspective, and spending time doing something else—playing an instrument, going to a museum, reading or listening to a great book—can make your endeavors of change less onerous and more a part of your overall life. Remember, the fullness of life makes it more important than even the individual goals we set and work so hard to achieve.

Meal 1 (choose 1 of the following):

- Large fruit plate of melon, grapes, and banana slices (swap out fruits per your preference) with 6 to 8 ounces 100% plain Greek yogurt, berries, and granola
- Frittata with cheese and your choice of vegetables
- 1½ cups cooked oatmeal, with sliced fruit

Meal 2 (choose 1 of the following):

- Turkey or chicken sandwich on 100% whole-wheat or whole-grain bread with lettuce, tomato, and cheese and a small green garden salad
- 6-ounce veggie burger on 100% whole-wheat or whole-grain bun with lettuce, tomato, and cheese and a small green garden salad

Meal 3 (choose 1 of the following):

- 6 ounces grilled or baked fish with squash or zucchini slices (3 to 5 ounces sliced chicken optional)
- 4 servings of cooked vegetables (spinach, black-eyed peas, sweet potato, and chickpeas)
- 2 slices whole-wheat or whole-grain pizza and a small green garden salad

Snacks (choose 3 snacks from below and eat them whenever you want during your feeding window):

- Loaded pepper slices (1 cup red bell pepper slices topped with ¼ cup warm black beans and 1 tablespoon guacamole)
- 1 cup fresh cherries
- 8 to 10 green or black olives
- Frozen banana slices (1 whole banana)
- 2 sticks fat-free or low-fat string cheese
- 1 large apple, sliced, sprinkled with cinnamon
- ¼ cup raw mixed nuts
- Watermelon cheese skewers (take 6 toothpicks and on each place 2 cubes watermelon and 1 cube (about the size of one die) feta cheese or your cheese of choice, and 1 slice cucumber)
- 10 to 15 baked sweet potato fries brushed with extra-virgin olive oil and sea salt
- 1 cup mixed fruit salad

Work It Out!

> ### *Exhaust Yourself*
>
> That burn and ache you feel in your muscles is a signal that you've worked as hard as possible and taken your muscles to full exhaustion. This is a state you want to reach—not all the time, but often enough so that you know what it means to bring yourself to exhaustion. Muscles give a bigger response when they've been worked maximally, so feel the burn and know that you've maximized your caloric burn and set yourself up for optimal muscle toning.

Beginner: Workout #6 (page 138)

Intermediate: Workout #6 (page 148)

Advanced: Workout #5 (page 157)

THE MORE YOU KNOW!

NATURAL APPETITE SUPPRESSANTS

Crunchy vegetables are a great way to suppress your appetite. Scientists don't know why the crunch triggers a sense of satiation, but anecdotal data strongly supports that it does. Here are some snacks you might try: carrots, celery, nuts, cucumbers, edamame, roasted chickpeas, kale chips, apples, pears, etc.

DAY 25

"Sometimes the biggest limits we face are those we set on ourselves."

Make today a day of extras. Push yourself to go the extra step in all that you do. The body transforms and improves when it is increasingly challenged. And while you might be doing what is suggested or expected of you, doing a little more can be what you need to stretch into this improvement zone. Today, add a little more to your exercise. For example, if you're jumping rope, do an extra 25 revolutions. Make your exercise sessions five to ten minutes longer than recommended. Eat your foods extra clean today and load up on water. Make this an A+ kind of day where you excel even beyond what is asked of you. It's important to know that even your best can be better.

Meal 1 (choose 1 of the following):

- 1 protein shake (350 calories or less)
- 1 fruit smoothie (350 calories or less)
- 1 grilled cheese sandwich made with 100% whole-wheat or whole-grain bread and organic cheese

Meal 2 (choose 1 of the following):

- 6 ounces grilled or baked halibut (or a fish of your preference)
- Large kale salad with nuts and/or shelled sunflower seeds, tomatoes, and orange slices

Meal 3 (choose 1 of the following):

- 6-ounce grilled or baked chicken breast with 2 servings of vegetables
- 6-ounce grilled or baked fish with 2 servings of vegetables
- 4 servings of cooked vegetables of your choice

Snacks (choose 3 snacks from below and eat them whenever you want during your feeding window):

- 1 cup fresh berries
- 20 raw almonds
- 15 walnuts
- ½ grapefruit
- ½ cup shelled or unshelled sunflower seeds
- 1 hard-boiled egg sprinkled with salt and choice of spices (pepper, paprika, etc.)
- ½ cucumber (8 to 10 slices) and 2 tablespoons hummus
- ½ cup raw or cooked vegetables
- ¼ cup peanuts, cashews, almonds, or pecans
- ¾ cup steamed edamame (in shell)

Work It Out!

Keep Your Workout Home

While it's typically effective and productive to work out in a gym, not everyone likes a gym atmosphere or can afford a membership. Sometimes, you just want to get a quick workout in without having to schlep to an outside facility. You can stay home and still get a very good workout with three simple tools: kettlebell, medicine ball, and resistance band.

Beginner: Rest

Intermediate: Rest

Advanced: Rest

THE MORE YOU KNOW!

SUGARMANIA!

The consumption of added sugar in the U.S. is out of control and its health consequence is being felt by millions. While most people think desserts and other sweet snacks are the major culprit, the truth is that sugar in liquid form is our biggest consumption. According to the USDA, sugary beverages like sodas, sports drinks, and energy drinks comprise an astounding 36 percent of the added sugar Americans take in daily. There's also evidence that it's more difficult to feel as full from a high-calorie sugary drink than it is from eating the same amount of calories via solid foods.

DAY 26

*"The heart is the engine that powers your body, so choose
clean foods to give it the highest octane fuel."*

Your body is a machine that needs to be fueled and pro-
tected and cared for with great attention and thought. Think of
your food as fuel. You want the cleanest, most nutrient-dense foods
that will nourish and satisfy you and taste great at the same time.
Make a mental connection between the food that you eat and what
it's doing to your body. If you're eating leafy green vegetables, think
about all of the fiber you're ingesting and how it is helping cleanse
your gastrointestinal tract. When eating your chicken sandwich,
think about the lean protein and how it is helping to build your
muscles. As you eat that cup of berries, think about all of the power-
ful antioxidants that will help neutralize those dangerous free
radicals lurking around that could cause disease. Food can be fun
and exciting, but never forget that it's your body's most important
fuel.

Meal 1 (choose 1 of the following):

- Fruit smoothie (350 calories or less)
- Protein shake (350 calories or less)

Meal 2 (choose 1 of the following):

- Turkey sandwich on 100% whole-wheat or whole-grain
  bread with 5 ounces turkey, with 1 ounce cheese (optional),
  tomato, lettuce, and organic mustard or clean mayonnaise
  (see recipe, page 222) and side serving of raw or cooked
  vegetables

- Large green garden salad with 2 tablespoons clean salad dressing (see recipes, pages 223–224) (3 to 5 ounces sliced chicken breast or fish optional)

Meal 3 (choose 1 of the following):

- 5-ounce veggie burger on 100% whole-wheat or whole-grain bun with lettuce, tomato, and onion with a medium green garden salad
- 5-ounce turkey burger on 100% whole-wheat or whole-grain bun with lettuce, tomato, and onion with a medium green garden salad
- 5-ounce chicken burger on 100% whole-wheat or whole-grain bun with lettuce, tomato, and onion with a medium green garden salad

Snacks (choose 3 snacks from below and eat them whenever you want during your feeding window):

- 2 dates stuffed with almonds (take out the pits and replace with 2 almonds)
- 3 tomato slices and fresh basil drizzled with extra-virgin olive oil
- 8 baby carrots with 2 tablespoons hummus
- 1 slice whole-wheat or whole-grain pita bread, cut into quarters, with 2 tablespoons hummus
- 10 cherries mixed with a handful of nuts (cashews, almonds, or walnuts)
- ½ cup shelled or unshelled pistachios
- 1 large apple, orange, or banana
- 2 small peaches
- 3 cups air-popped popcorn (light seasoning)
- 1 cup mixed fruit salad

Work It Out!

> ### *Lift, then Run*
>
> It's okay to sometimes do cardio and resistance training in the same workout; it might help you reach your goals faster. Try doing the resistance portion first, followed by your cardio work. This can maximize your muscle training, and the cardio can help provide a stretch as well as endurance work.

Beginner: Workout #6 (page 138)

Intermediate: Workout #6 (page 148)

Advanced: Workout #7 (page 159)

THE MORE YOU KNOW!

BUILD MUSCLE WITH FOOD

Protein is the building block of muscle. For most people, consuming between 65 to 80 grams of protein each day is enough to replenish protein stores and have extra to help build bigger, stronger muscles. Eat as much natural protein as possible in the form of food. Chicken, turkey, and fish are great sources of lean protein without costing a lot of calories. Legumes, including beans, peas, lentils, and peanuts, are a great source of nonanimal proteins. If you're consuming protein supplements in the form of shakes or smoothies, make sure you read the label for the amount of sugar and calories each scoop contains.

DAY 27

"Beauty sitting right in front of you is easy to miss when you're too busy to slow down and open your eyes."

Slow down and take it all in. Sometimes we're going so fast, rushing from one thing to the next, that we don't take the time to truly enjoy and appreciate moments. Remember that being present and alert and soaking in even the smallest of details, like the color of the flowers in your neighbor's yard, can go a long way to relieving stress and giving your life and purpose greater context. The urgency to get done what's on our task list unfortunately makes us vulnerable to ignoring so many things that can bring value to our lives. Executing and achieving are great and commendable, but every so often, look up toward the sky before going into your house at night. The stars are always magical and humbling and mysterious. They can also help align your emotional and psychological axes and keep them in perspective.

Meal 1 (choose 1 of the following):

- Turkey bacon, egg, and cheese sandwich on 100% whole-wheat or whole-grain bread with a side of fruit
- 1½ cups cooked oatmeal with a side of fruit (honey and cinnamon allowed)
- 2 scrambled eggs with cheese and/or veggies and 1 slice 100% whole-wheat or whole-grain toast

Meal 2 (choose 1 of the following):

- 1½ cups whole-wheat or whole-grain spaghetti with sun-dried tomatoes (3 to 5 ounces grilled chicken strips or fish optional)

- 1½ cups soup (noncreamy)
- Large green garden salad with 2 tablespoons clean salad dressing (see recipes, pages 223–224)

Meal 3 (choose 1 of the following):

- 4 servings cooked vegetables (corn, zucchini, black beans, and watercress) with ½ cup cooked quinoa or brown rice
- 6 ounces grilled or baked fish with 2 servings of vegetables
- 6-ounce turkey burger on 100% whole-wheat or whole-grain bun with cheese, lettuce, and tomato and a green garden salad

Snacks (choose 3 snacks from below and eat them whenever you want during your feeding window):

- 8 to 10 green or black olives
- ½ cup organic fat-free or low-fat cottage cheese
- ¼ cup wasabi peas
- 1 cup mixed fruit salad
- 10 walnut halves and 1 sliced kiwi
- 1 cup watermelon and red onion salad
- 1 sliced red pepper with 2 tablespoons hummus
- ½ cup black bean dip and 8 veggie sticks (carrots or celery)
- 1 small baked sweet potato
- 8 olives stuffed with 1 tablespoon feta or blue cheese

Work It Out!

Mini Workouts Make a Difference

Workouts don't always have to be long to make a difference. Short, intense workouts can still burn a lot of calories and give your body a challenge that can produce results. A 10- or 15-minute workout can be done quickly and effectively and can be completed right at home or even during a break at work.

Beginner: Workout #7 (page 139)

Intermediate: Workout #7 (page 149)

Advanced: Workout #7 (page 159)

THE MORE YOU KNOW!

THE DIRTY DOZEN

Despite what many think, organic doesn't always mean healthier. In most cases you don't need organic produce, but if you want organic, spend your money wisely by choosing organic for those fruits and veggies with edible skin or peel. Consider these:

Apples	Peaches
Celery	Pears
Cherries	Potatoes
Grapes	Spinach
Lettuce	Strawberries
Nectarines	Peppers

DAY 28

*"A positive attitude can spread like a mutated virus
with no medication to stop it."*

Spread your enthusiasm, because success can be contagious. When you are enthusiastic and others see that, they too are more inclined to be enthusiastic. When you are dour and skeptical, others around you will respond accordingly. Getting into a positive space and staying there can take a lot of effort, as there are so many distractions that can try to pull you into a negative space. You can be a lightning rod for positivity by doing even the simplest things, such as speaking to someone as you get on the elevator or offering to buy someone a cup of coffee. You will be amazed at how the smallest of gestures can have such a significant impact on those around you, mostly because we have been conditioned not to expect niceties from others in our fast-paced lives. It's also important to surround yourself with people who have a positive outlook and want to be in a better space. It's easy for others to drag you down, people who constantly want to unload negative emotions or viewpoints and take even the best situations and dissect them until they find a thin line of negativity to grasp and not let go. We all have met these people, and in some cases we have no choice but to interact with them. But when you can control your environment and the company you keep, seek those who are positive and enthusiastic and optimistic that good things can and will happen.

Meal 1 (choose 1 of the following):

- Fruit smoothie (350 calories or less)
- Tropical smoothie bowl (1½ cups fruit: pulse banana, mango, pineapple, and almond milk until smooth and thick; top with blueberries, kiwi, and peaches)

Meal 2 (choose 1 of the following):

- Turkey or chicken sandwich on 100% whole-wheat or whole-grain bread with lettuce, tomato, and cheese and a small green garden salad
- 6-ounce veggie burger on 100% whole-wheat or whole-grain bun with lettuce, tomato, and cheese and a small green garden salad

Meal 3 (choose 1 of the following):

- 6-ounce turkey burger on 100% whole-wheat or whole-grain bun with tomato, lettuce, and cheese and a baked or mashed sweet potato and cauliflower or green beans
- 1½ cups soup (tomato, bean, chickpea, or lentil) with a small green garden salad

Snacks (choose 3 snacks from below and eat them whenever you want during your feeding window):

- 20 seedless grapes with 10 almonds or cashews
- Kale chips (½ cup raw kale, stems removed, baked with 1 teaspoon olive oil at 400°F until crisp)
- 1 hard-boiled egg sprinkled with salt and choice of spices (pepper, paprika, etc.)
- ½ cucumber (8 to 10 slices) and 2 tablespoons hummus
- ½ cup raw or cooked vegetables
- ¼ cup walnuts (or peanuts, cashews, almonds, or pecans)
- 1 cup steamed shelled edamame

- 10 cherry tomatoes sprinkled with salt, pepper, and vinaigrette
- 3 ounces fresh cooked turkey breast slices and raw veggies or, if deli turkey slices, make sure it's nitrites/nitrates-free, no antibiotics, no artificial flavors, no preservatives

Work It Out!

> ### Radical Change
>
> Your body can be lulled into complacency by doing the same workouts repetitively. Every 3 weeks, make some radical changes. When you work out, the order of exercises, the location of your workout—change it all up for a week. This will not only stimulate different muscles but also keep your mind fresh.

Beginner: Rest

Intermediate: Rest

Advanced: Rest

THE MORE YOU KNOW!

ADVANTAGES OF LIGHTER, MORE FREQUENT MEALS

Better stabilization of blood sugars throughout the day

Even distribution of calories throughout the day

Fewer cravings between meals

Reduction of cortisol levels (high levels of cortisol hormone have been shown to be correlated with increased abdominal fat)

DAY 29

> *"A closed mind and a closed palate are like living*
> *in a house without windows."*

It's easy to get into a rut of doing the same things the same way, when life becomes less exciting and more mundane. Keep an open mind and be willing to try new things. Whether it's a new type of cuisine or a different type of exercise or stress-relieving method, be willing to experiment with a positive attitude that something good will come of it. The hectic nature of the world we live in lulls us into a type of behavioral conditioning where we are less willing to deviate from routine. This puts you in a box; while you might be comfortable knowing the walls that surround you, there is little opportunity or desire to venture into unfamiliar territory that might harbor new opportunities that you find exciting and beneficial. Do something completely different today, whether it's a new food that you've never tried or an exercise you've been too hesitant to add to your workout. Don't go into it with the mindset that you probably won't like it; rather take on a positive attitude that this is something you are willing and likely to enjoy. If you do this just a couple of times a week, think about all the new things you'll be adding to your world and the infinite possibilities before you.

Meal 1 (choose 1 of the following):

- 2-egg broccoli and cheese omelet
- 2-egg asparagus-mushroom frittata
- Fruit smoothie (350 calories or less)

Meal 2 (choose 1 of the following):

- Tuna salad sandwich on 100% whole-wheat or whole-grain bread with lettuce, ½ cup raw carrots, and hummus
- Chicken sandwich on 100% whole-wheat or whole-grain bread with tomato, lettuce, clean mayo (see recipe, page 222), and 1 ounce cheese (optional) with a small green garden salad

Meal 3 (choose 1 of the following):

- Large green garden salad with 2 tablespoons clean salad dressing (see recipes, pages 223–224) (3 to 5 ounces sliced chicken breast or fish optional)
- 2 cups soup (chicken, lentil, bean, or butternut squash)

Snacks (choose 3 snacks from below and eat them whenever you want during your feeding window):

- ¼ cup mushrooms marinated in extra-virgin olive oil, salt, and pepper
- 4 clean turkey meatballs (1-inch diameter)
- ¼ cup baked apple chips
- ⅓ cup egg salad made with clean mayonnaise (see mayonnaise recipe, page 222)
- ⅔ cup cauliflower with 2 tablespoons hummus
- 1 nonfat mozzarella cheese stick with 1 small apple
- Sliced tomatoes with a pinch of pepper and/or salt and olive oil
- Ten 100% whole-wheat or whole-grain pretzels
- 1 large beefsteak tomato slice and 1 tablespoon feta cheese
- ½ cup cucumber slices and organic vinaigrette dressing

Work It Out!

> ## *Define Your Goals*
>
> On a piece of paper or in your phone, write down specific goals you would like to achieve. Make sure the benchmarks are clear and precise and measurable. Keep track of your progress on a daily basis, making sure you are sticking to the plan and hitting your milestones. Your goal sheet is an important yardstick as well as a motivational tool.

Beginner: Workout #7 (page 139)

Intermediate: Workout #7 (page 149)

Advanced: Workout #7 (page 159)

THE MORE YOU KNOW!

SIMPLE BMI CHART

$$BMI = Weight\ (kg)\ /\ Height\ (m) \times Height\ (m)$$

BMI	Weight Status
Below 18.5	Underweight
18.6–24.9	Normal
25–29.9	Overweight
30 and above	Obese

DAY 30

*"Regardless of what you accomplish, always consider
yourself a work in progress, for this humility
will allow you to accomplish even more."*

If you were printing out a view of your life, choose your
printer's landscape option instead of portrait so that you have a
broader view. Now that you have taken this journey, it's important
to reflect on not just the milestones you reached or missed, but
what you learned about yourself, your relationship to food, your
mental approach to change, and how doing things differently can
make you feel better and more inspired. It's easy to get stuck thinking about what's right in front of you rather than stepping back
and taking a long view about where you've been and what lies ahead.
The landscape view gives you this perspective. The lessons you've
learned and changes you've made are meant to be a blueprint for
how you live the rest of your life. It's unrealistic to expect you to
eat perfectly or limit yourself to thirty foods forever. Undoubtedly,
you will eat processed foods that you've avoided in the last month.
However, one of the most valuable lessons of this journey has been
to show you what you can actually do when you put your mind to
it and stick to the plan. You now know that you have the ability to
make corrections and tough decisions if necessary and you can rein
yourself in if you are going too far astray. "Everything in modera-
tion" is more than just a saying, it is an effective way to keep balance in your life without feeling like you need to obsess about
whether everything you do is right or wrong. Maintain as many of
the good habits you've picked up along the journey as possible,
and this new way of living will make a *NEW YOU*!

Meal 1 (choose 1 of the following):

- Avocado spread on 2 slices 100% whole-wheat or whole-grain bread with 2 slices turkey bacon
- 2 scrambled eggs (cheese and diced vegetables optional) with 2 slices turkey bacon

Meal 2 (choose 1 of the following):

- Turkey sandwich on 100% whole-wheat or whole-grain bread with lettuce, tomato, and cheese and a small green garden salad
- Large green garden salad with 2 tablespoons clean salad dressing (see recipes, pages 223–224) (3 to 5 ounces sliced chicken breast or fish optional)

Meal 3 (choose 1 of the following):

- 6-ounce grilled or baked chicken breast with 2 servings of vegetables
- 6-ounce grilled or baked fish with 2 servings of vegetables
- 4 servings of cooked vegetables of your choice

Snacks (choose 3 snacks from below and eat them whenever you want during your feeding window):

- Kale chips (½ cup raw kale, stems removed, baked with 1 teaspoon olive oil at 400°F until crisp)
- 1 cup fresh berries
- 20 raw almonds
- 15 walnuts
- ½ grapefruit
- ½ cup shelled or unshelled sunflower seeds
- Fresh fruit popsicle (made only from freshly squeezed juice and frozen into cubes)
- 2 slices grilled pineapple

- ½ cup banana slices and 1 tablespoon organic peanut butter
- 15 to 20 unroasted peanuts

Work It Out!

Be Consistent

One of the best ways to make progress in your workouts is to be consistent. Starting and stopping a program keeps you stuck in the same place. Even if you aren't enthusiastic about your workout or you don't think you can do all of it, at least do some of it. Just doing whatever you can keeps you on track.

Beginner: Workout #7 (page 139)

Intermediate: Workout #7 (page 149)

Advanced: Workout #7 (page 159)

THE MORE YOU KNOW!

DISEASES AND HEALTH CONDITIONS RELATED TO OBESITY

Coronary heart disease

Dyslipidemia (for example, high LDL cholesterol, low HDL cholesterol, or high levels of triglycerides)

Gallbladder disease

Hypertension (high blood pressure)

Osteoarthritis

Sleep apnea and respiratory problems

Some cancers (endometrial, breast, and colon)

III

The WORKOUTS

5

THE WORKOUT PLANS

BEGINNER WORKOUTS

These workouts are designed for people who are just beginning their fitness journey or who have been relatively sedentary for a while and want to get back into the game. The most important concept around these workouts is patience. You might not be able to complete an entire workout as written, and that's perfectly fine. What's most important is that you do the best you can. Every 10 to 14 days you should see some improvements, whether it's in your ability to execute the exercise maneuvers, stamina, strength, or increased muscle tone.

The workouts have been constructed so that they are listed in increasing complexity and difficulty. Once you have mastered a particular workout, feel free to move up to the next one. It's unlikely you will be able to complete the new workout as effectively as you did the previous one, but eventually you will come to master the new workout too.

Everyone brings with them different levels of fitness, physical capabilities, and goals. If you find that one exercise is more troublesome for you compared to another one, go ahead and swap it out and do another one from the list of exercises from your workout track. Flexibility is an important component to your exercise regimen, as there is no one-size-fits-all. Modifications that allow you to do the best you can and keep you motivated to stick to the program are what you should be embracing.

Just because you start as a beginner doesn't mean you have to stay a beginner. The goal is that as your fitness level improves, you will be able to tackle more difficult exercises, so don't be afraid to experiment and move up to an intermediate exercise. Remember that those workouts are also ordered in increasing difficulty, so start with Workout #1 and then progress from there.

Super Sets are done at the end of the workout. This is a quick circuit of all of the exercises that you performed during the workout. The rest breaks between the exercises are designed to be shorter so that you spend considerably more time in the active interval rather than the rest phase.

WORKOUT #1

Total Workout Time: 15 minutes

- 11,000 steps over the course of the day
- 5 staircases over the course of the day (1 staircase is considered to be a trip up and down)

The following exercises should be done consecutively in a fashion such that they are all completed within the allotted time given. Don't break up the exercises by doing them at different times of the day. Do the best you can to complete them as written.

- 35 seconds of **Marching High Knees** followed by 35 seconds of rest—repeat 3 times
- 35 seconds of **Step-Ups** followed by 35 seconds of rest—repeat 3 times
- 35 seconds of **Jump Rope** followed by 35 seconds of rest—repeat 3 times

Super Set

- 35 seconds of **Marching High Knees**
- 20 seconds of **Rest**
- 35 seconds of **Step-Ups**
- 20 seconds of **Rest**
- 35 seconds of **Jump Rope**

WORKOUT #2

Total Workout Time: 20 minutes

- 12,000 steps over the course of the day
- 7 staircases throughout the day (1 staircase is considered to be a trip up and down)

The following exercises should be done consecutively in a fashion such that they are all completed within the allotted time given. Don't break up the exercises by doing them at different times of the day. Do the best you can to complete them as written.

- 45 seconds of **Jog Punches** followed by 35 seconds of rest—repeat 4 times
- 45 seconds of **Steam Engines** followed by 35 seconds of rest—repeat 4 times
- 45 seconds of **Squats** followed by 35 seconds of rest—repeat 4 times

Super Set

- 45 seconds of **Jog Punches**
- 25 seconds of **Rest**
- 45 seconds of **Steam Engines**
- 25 seconds of **Rest**
- 45 seconds of **Squats**

WORKOUT #3

Total Workout Time: 15 minutes

- 13,000 steps over the course of the day

The following exercises should be done consecutively in a fashion such that they are all completed within the allotted time given. Don't break up the exercises by doing them at different times of the day. Do the best you can to complete them as written.

- 8 consecutive **Staircases** in less than 90 seconds (1 staircase is considered to be a trip up and down)
- 60 seconds of **Jump Rope** followed by 45 seconds of rest—repeat 3 times
- 60 seconds of **Star Jumps** followed by 45 seconds of rest—repeat 3 times

Super Set

- 1 **Staircase** in less than 10 seconds
- 10 seconds of **Rest**
- 60 seconds of **Jump Rope**
- 25 seconds of rest
- 60 seconds of **Star Jumps**

WORKOUT #4

Total Workout Time: 15 minutes

- 14,000 steps over the course of the day
- 10 staircases completed at once or throughout the day (1 staircase is considered to be a trip up and down)

The following exercises should be done consecutively in a fashion such that they are all completed within the allotted time given. Don't break up the exercises by doing them at different times of the day. Do the best you can to complete them as written.

- 60 seconds of **Steam Engines** followed by 45 seconds of rest—repeat 2 times
- 60 seconds of **Jump Rope** followed by 45 seconds of rest—repeat 2 times
- 60 seconds of **Squats** followed by 45 seconds of rest—repeat 2 times

Super Set

- 60 seconds of **Steam Engines**
- 30 seconds of **Rest**
- 60 seconds of **Jump Rope**
- 30 seconds of **Rest**
- 60 seconds of **Squats**

WORKOUT #5

Total Workout Time: 25 minutes

- 11,000 steps to be completed throughout the day

The following exercises should be done consecutively in a fashion such that they are all completed within the allotted time given. Don't break up the exercises by doing them at different times of the day. Do the best you can to complete them as written.

- 60 seconds of **Marching High Knees** followed by 30 seconds of rest—repeat 3 times
- 60 seconds of **Squats** followed by 30 seconds of rest—repeat 3 times
- 60 seconds of **Jog Punches** followed by 30 seconds of rest—repeat 3 times
- 60 seconds of **Step-Ups** followed by 30 seconds of rest—repeat 3 times

Super Set

- 60 seconds of **Marching High Knees**
- 20 seconds of **Rest**
- 60 seconds of **Squats**
- 20 seconds of **Rest**
- 60 seconds of **Jog Punches**
- 20 seconds of **Rest**
- 60 seconds of **Step-Ups**

WORKOUT #6

Total Workout Time: 20 minutes

- 60 seconds of **Step-Ups**, followed by 30 seconds of running in place, followed by 35 seconds of rest—repeat 2 times

- 60 seconds of **Squats**, followed by 30 seconds of running in place, followed by 35 seconds of rest—repeat 2 times

- 60 seconds of **Jumping Jacks**, followed by 30 seconds of running in place, followed by 35 seconds of rest—repeat 2 times

- 60 seconds of **Steam Engines**, followed by 30 seconds of running in place, followed by 35 seconds of rest— repeat 2 times

Super Set

- 30 seconds of **Step-Ups**
- 10 seconds of **Rest**
- 30 seconds of **Squats**
- 15 seconds of **Rest**
- 30 seconds of **Jumping Jacks**
- 20 seconds of **Rest**
- 30 seconds of **Steam Engines**

WORKOUT #7

Total Workout Time: 30 minutes

This is a circuit workout that consists of six exercises. You need to set aside enough time to do the entire circuit *twice*. Staying on time is critical to the success of this circuit, so make sure you are following the time allotments as written as well as you can.

- 45 seconds of **Star Jumps**, followed by 45 seconds of running in place, followed by 45 seconds of rest
- 45 seconds of **Jog Punches**, followed by 45 seconds of running in place, followed by 45 seconds of rest
- 45 seconds of **Staircases**, followed by 45 seconds of running in place, followed by 45 seconds of rest
- 45 seconds of **Marching High Knees**, followed by 45 seconds of squats, followed by 45 seconds of rest
- 45 seconds of **Squats**, followed by 45 seconds of running in place, followed by 45 seconds of rest
- 45 seconds of **Jumping Rope**, followed by 45 seconds of rest

REPEAT ENTIRE CIRCUIT.

INTERMEDIATE WORKOUTS

This is a timed workout, and the exercises should be performed in a consecutive fashion. If you aren't able to complete the entire active interval of the workout without stopping, don't worry. Stop when you need to, finish the rest period, then go back to the active period as specified. For example, if you're supposed to have an active phase of 40 seconds and a rest phase of 35 seconds and you can only do 25 seconds of the active phase, go ahead and begin your rest period early. So instead of resting for 35 seconds, you will rest for 50 seconds. The key, however, is to not rest longer than that and to begin your next active phase on time. These workouts are most effective when you stick to the timed interval sequences and do not extend the rest portion too much beyond what has been allotted.

If you want to change the order of the exercises, feel free to do so, but keep in mind the body parts that are being worked. While it will not always be possible to give a specific muscle group complete rest from one exercise to another, definitely try your best to separate their usage.

Super Sets are done at the end of the workout. This is a quick circuit of all of the exercises that you performed during the workout. The rest breaks between the exercises are designed to be shorter so that you spend considerably more time in the active interval rather than the rest phase.

WORKOUT #1

Total Workout Time: 15 minutes

- 40 seconds of **Ice Skaters** followed by 35 seconds of rest—repeat 3 times
- 40 seconds of **Butt Kicks** followed by 35 seconds of rest—repeat 3 times
- 40 seconds of **Lunges** followed by 35 seconds of rest—repeat 3 times

Super Set

- 40 seconds of **Ice Skaters**
- 15 seconds of **Rest**
- 40 seconds of **Butt Kicks**
- 15 seconds of **Rest**
- 40 seconds of **Lunges**

WORKOUT #2

Total Workout Time: 20 minutes

- 45 seconds of **Line Hops** followed by 35 seconds of rest—repeat 4 times
- 45 seconds of **Planking** followed by 35 seconds of rest—repeat 4 times
- 45 seconds of **Running High Knees** followed by 35 seconds of rest—repeat 4 times

Super Set

- 45 seconds of **Line Hops**
- 15 seconds of **Rest**
- 45 seconds of **Planking**
- 15 seconds of **Rest**
- 45 seconds of **Running High Knees**

WORKOUT #3

Total Workout Time: 15 minutes

- 45 seconds of **Modified Grasshopper** followed by 35 seconds of rest—repeat 3 times
- 45 seconds of **Cycling** (high-speed sprint) followed by 35 seconds of rest—repeat 3 times
- 45 seconds of **Plank Jacks** followed by 35 seconds of rest—repeat 3 times

Super Set

- 45 seconds of **Modified Grasshopper**
- 15 seconds of **Rest**
- 45 seconds of **Cycling** (high-speed sprint)
- 15 seconds of **Rest**
- 45 seconds of **Plank Jacks**

WORKOUT #4

Total Workout Time: 25 minutes

- 45 seconds of **Squat Jumps** followed by 35 seconds of rest—repeat 3 times
- 45 seconds of **Line Hops** followed by 35 seconds of rest—repeat 3 times
- 45 seconds of **Planking** followed by 35 seconds of rest—repeat 3 times
- 45 seconds of **Butt Kicks** followed by 35 seconds of rest—repeat 3 times

Super Set

- 45 seconds of **Squat Jumps**
- 15 seconds of **Rest**
- 45 seconds of **Line Hops**
- 15 seconds of **Rest**
- 45 seconds of **Planking**
- 15 seconds of **Rest**
- 45 seconds of **Butt Kicks**

WORKOUT #5

Total Workout Time: 25 minutes

- 60 seconds of **Ice Skaters** followed by 40 seconds of rest—repeat 3 times
- 60 seconds of **Plank Jacks** followed by 40 seconds of rest—repeat 3 times
- 60 seconds of **High Knees** followed by 40 seconds of rest—repeat 3 times
- 60 seconds of **Line Hops** followed by 40 seconds of rest—repeat 3 times

Super Set

- 60 seconds of **Ice Skaters**
- 20 seconds of **Rest**
- 60 seconds of **Plank Jacks**
- 20 seconds of **Rest**
- 60 seconds of **High Knees**
- 20 seconds of **Rest**
- 60 seconds of **Line Hops**

WORKOUT #6

This is a circuit workout that consists of six exercises. You need to set aside enough time to do the entire circuit *twice*. Staying on time is critical to the success of this circuit, so make sure you are following the time allotments as written as well as you can.

Total Workout Time: 30 minutes

- 45 seconds of **Butt Kicks**, followed by 45 seconds of running in place, followed by 45 seconds of rest
- 45 seconds of **Planking**, followed by 45 seconds of running in place, followed by 45 seconds of rest
- 45 seconds of **Squat Jumps**, followed by 45 seconds of running in place, followed by 45 seconds of rest
- 45 seconds of **Line Hops**, followed by 45 seconds of running in place, followed by 45 seconds of rest
- 45 seconds of **Planking**, followed by 45 seconds of running in place, followed by 45 seconds of rest
- 45 seconds of **Running High Knees**, followed by 45 seconds of rest

REPEAT ENTIRE CIRCUIT.

WORKOUT #7

This is a circuit workout that consists of six exercises. You need to set aside enough time to do the entire circuit *twice*. Staying on time is critical to the success of this circuit, so make sure you are following the time allotments as written as well as you can.

Total Workout Time: 30 minutes

- 60 seconds of **Ice Skaters**, followed by 30 seconds of jumping jacks, followed by 45 seconds of rest
- 60 seconds of **Plank Jacks**, followed by 30 seconds of running in place, followed by 45 seconds of rest
- 60 seconds of **Lunges**, followed by 30 seconds of running in place, followed by 45 seconds of rest
- 60 seconds of **Cycling** (high-speed sprints), followed by 30 seconds of jumping jacks, followed by 45 seconds of rest
- 60 seconds of **Planking**, followed by 30 seconds of running in place, followed by 45 seconds of rest
- 60 seconds of **Squat Jumps**, followed by 30 seconds of jumping jacks, followed by 45 seconds of rest

REPEAT ENTIRE CIRCUIT.

ADVANCED WORKOUTS

These workouts are designed to be challenging. The movements, effort required, and complexity of the programs are set for someone who is more advanced, with greater than normal stamina. Recovery is definitely important for this category, so don't attempt to do these workouts more than two days consecutively. In fact, you might even consider doing an advanced workout day followed by an intermediate or beginner program day to give yourself some relative rest.

This is a timed workout, and the exercises should be performed in a consecutive fashion. If you aren't able to complete the entire active interval of the workout without stopping, don't worry. Stop when you need to, finish the rest period, then go back to the active period as specified. For example, if you're supposed to have an active phase of 40 seconds and a rest phase of 35 seconds and you can only do 25 seconds of the active phase, go ahead and begin your rest period early. So instead of resting for 35 seconds, you will rest for 50 seconds. The key, however, is to not rest longer than that and to begin your next active phase on time. These workouts are most effective when you stick to the timed interval sequences and do not extend the rest portion too much beyond what has been allotted.

If you want to change the order of the exercises, feel free to do so, but keep in mind the body parts that are being worked. While it will not always be possible to give a specific muscle group complete rest from one exercise to another, definitely try your best to separate their usage.

Super Sets are done at the end of the workout. This is a quick circuit of all of the exercises that you performed during the workout.

The rest breaks between the exercises are designed to be shorter so that you spend considerably more time in the active interval rather than the rest phase.

WORKOUT #1

Total Workout Time: 15 minutes

- 35 seconds of **Mountain Climbers** followed by 35 seconds of rest—repeat 3 times
- 35 seconds of **Tuck Jumps** followed by 35 seconds of rest—repeat 3 times
- 35 seconds of **Kettlebell Swings** followed by 35 seconds of rest—repeat 3 times

Super Set

- 35 seconds of **Mountain Climbers**
- 15 seconds of **Rest**
- 35 seconds of **Tuck Jumps**
- 15 seconds of **Rest**
- 35 seconds of **Kettlebell Swings**

WORKOUT #2

Total Workout Time: 20 minutes

- 35 seconds of **Burpees** followed by 35 seconds of rest—repeat 3 times
- 35 seconds of **Frog Jumps** followed by 35 seconds of rest—repeat 3 times
- 35 seconds of **Ab Twists** followed by 35 seconds of rest—repeat 3 times

Super Set

- 35 seconds of **Burpees**
- 20 seconds of **Rest**
- 35 seconds of **Frog Jumps**
- 20 seconds of **Rest**
- 35 seconds of **Ab Twists**

WORKOUT #3

Total Workout Time: 20 minutes

- 45 seconds of **Rowing** followed by 35 seconds of rest—repeat 4 times
- 45 seconds of **Sprinting** followed by 35 seconds of rest—repeat 4 times
- 35 seconds of **Box Jumps** followed by 35 seconds of rest—repeat 4 times

Super Set

- 45 seconds of **Rowing**
- 25 seconds of **Rest**
- 45 seconds of **Sprinting**
- 25 seconds of **Rest**
- 35 seconds of **Box Jumps**

WORKOUT #4

Total Workout Time: 20 minutes

- 40 seconds of **Jumping Lunges** followed by 35 seconds of rest—repeat 3 times
- 40 seconds of **Kettlebell Swings** followed by 35 seconds of rest—repeat 3 times
- 40 seconds of **Tuck Jumps** followed by 35 seconds of rest—repeat 3 times
- 40 seconds of **Sprinting** followed by 35 seconds of rest—repeat 3 times

Super Set

- 40 seconds of **Jumping Lunges**
- 25 seconds of **Rest**
- 40 seconds of **Kettlebell Swings**
- 25 seconds of **Rest**
- 40 seconds of **Tuck Jumps**
- 25 seconds of **Rest**
- 40 seconds of **Sprinting**

WORKOUT #5

Total Workout Time: 20 minutes

- 40 seconds of **Mountain Climbers** followed by 35 seconds of rest—repeat 3 times
- 40 seconds of **Frog Jumps** followed by 35 seconds of rest—repeat 3 times
- 40 seconds of **Ab Twists** followed by 35 seconds of rest—repeat 3 times
- 40 seconds of **Burpees** followed by 35 seconds of rest—repeat 3 times

Super Set

- 40 seconds of **Mountain Climbers**
- 25 seconds of **Rest**
- 40 seconds of **Frog Jumps**
- 25 seconds of **Rest**
- 40 seconds of **Ab Twists**
- 25 seconds of **Rest**
- 40 seconds of **Burpees**

WORKOUT #6

This is a circuit workout that consists of six exercises. You need to set aside enough time to do the entire circuit *twice*. Staying on time is critical to the success of this circuit, so make sure you are following the time allotments as written as well as you can.

Total Workout Time: 25 minutes

- 45 seconds of **Sprinting**, followed by 30 seconds of jumping jacks, followed by 45 seconds of rest
- 45 seconds of **Jumping Lunges**, followed by 30 seconds of running in place, followed by 45 seconds of rest
- 45 seconds of **Ab Twists**, followed by 30 seconds of jumping jacks, followed by 45 seconds of rest
- 45 seconds of **Rowing** (high speed), followed by 30 seconds of running in place, followed by 45 seconds of rest
- 45 seconds of **Box Jumps**, followed by 30 seconds of jumping jacks, followed by 45 seconds of rest
- 45 seconds of **Kettlebell Swings**, followed by 30 seconds of running in place, followed by 45 seconds of rest

REPEAT ENTIRE CIRCUIT.

WORKOUT #7

This is a circuit workout that consists of six exercises. You need to set aside enough time to do the entire circuit *twice*. Staying on time is critical to the success of this circuit, so make sure you are following the time allotments as written as well as you can.

Total Workout Time: 30 minutes

- 60 seconds of **AB Twists**, followed by 30 seconds of running in place, followed by 45 seconds of rest
- 60 seconds of **Mountain Climbers**, followed by 30 seconds of running in place, followed by 45 seconds of rest
- 60 seconds of **Kettlebell Swings**, followed by 30 seconds of running in place, followed by 45 seconds of rest
- 60 seconds of **Tuck Jumps**, followed by 30 seconds of running in place, followed by 45 seconds of rest
- 60 seconds of **AB Twists**, followed by 30 seconds of running in place, followed by 45 seconds of rest
- 60 seconds of **Frog Jumps**, followed by 30 seconds of running in place, followed by 45 seconds of rest

REPEAT ENTIRE CIRCUIT.

6

EXERCISE INSTRUCTIONS

BEGINNER

HIGH KNEES (MARCHING)

JUMPING ROPE

SQUATS

STEAM ENGINES

JOG PUNCHES

JUMPING JACKS

WALKING

STAR JUMPS

STEP-UPS

STAIRS

HIGH KNEES (MARCHING)

This body-weight exercise is perfect to work
your cardiovascular system as well as toning
your lower extremities and core. Not only will
this help strengthen your body, but it will also
create very good caloric burn. Try to perform
this exercise continuously within a defined
period of time (15 seconds, 30 seconds, 45
seconds, and so on). Form matters, and push
yourself so that your heart rate kicks up into
another gear.

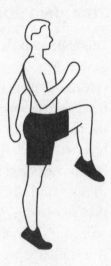

HOW TO

1. Stand up straight with your feet shoulder-width apart and
your feet pointing forward.

2. Place your arms at a 90-degree angle by your sides, just above
your waist with your hands balled into fists.

3. Drive your right knee up just above your waist while at the
same time pumping your left arm up in the air and your right arm
back—marching formation.

4. Alternate knees and pump your arms in the opposite orientation.

5. As your knees come up, be sure to engage (tighten or contract) your abdominal muscles to work your core.

JUMPING ROPE

This childhood exercise is an oldie but goodie. Muscle toning and a cardiovascular challenge occur at the same time. Jumping rope can be done various ways to change up your workout and to increase the challenge to your body. If you don't have a rope, you can use what's called an "air rope"—pretend that you have a rope and still move your hands accordingly. Pace yourself. If you need to start out by doing the exercise for a short amount of time (5 to 15 seconds), don't worry about it. It's always better to start slowly and build up your stamina rather than try to do too much too fast. As your comfort and skill level improve, try different jumps such as jumping on one leg or double jumping, which means turning the rope twice under your feet while doing a single jump.

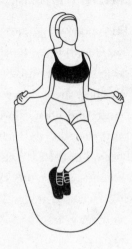

HOW TO

1. Place your hands level or slightly above your hips while holding the rope.

2. Rotate your wrists forward to swing the rope behind you and up over your head.

3. With your feet either together or slightly spread apart, jump while the rope is working its way up behind you. As you get more advanced, try jumping on one foot or alternating feet.

4. Repeat the turning and jumping sequence.

SQUATS

This maneuver is considered to be a compound full-body exercise that works several muscles of the body, including the thighs (quadriceps), buttocks (gluteus maximus), hamstrings, hips, and core. We do squats many times a day in our normal movement, whether it's getting in and out of a car, sitting on a toilet, standing up from the side of the bed, or standing up out of a chair. While bodybuilders and weightlifters use this exercise to improve strength and performance, it remains extremely beneficial for even the casual exerciser. As your strength and stability improve, you might try doing the squat with light dumbbells in your hands to add to the resistance and work of the exercise.

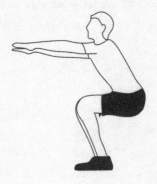

HOW TO

1. Stand with your feet shoulder-width apart or slightly wider.

2. Your feet should be facing forward and your chest held up and out.

3. Keep your torso erect and sit down as if sitting in a chair and stop when you reach parallel. If you want to do a more advanced squat and you don't have any joint or back problems, you might dip a little lower, to just beneath parallel. Keep your hands stretched out in front of you approximately chest high.

4. Hold your squat position for 3 seconds, then come back up. Stand for 2 seconds, then squat again.

STEAM ENGINES

Steam engines are also called "standing crunches." They work many muscles, primarily the abdominals and quadriceps. They also work the muscles that run down the outside of the legs—hip flexors. Many call this exercise a "standing crunch" due to how intensely it works and tightens the core. Make no mistake: while your abs are shredding, you're still sending a big jolt to your cardiovascular system, which heats up your calorie burning and trims the fat.

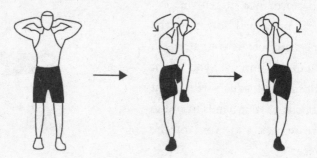

HOW TO

1. Stand tall with your feet shoulder-width apart. Clasp your hands behind your head with elbows forward and in line with your shoulders.

2. Do these two things at the same time: raise your left knee up and bring your right elbow (hands still clasped behind your head) toward your knee, touching it if you can.

3. Once you complete this movement, bring your leg back down and your head back up. Then repeat the same movement with the opposite leg and arm (right knee up with left elbow touching it).

Exercise Variation: If you have physical limitations, you can still do this exercise. Instead of clasping your hands behind your head, put your arms in a 90-degree angle at your side with your hands balled into fists and your forearms parallel to the ground. Take your right elbow across your body and at the same time lift your left knee. Try to touch your elbow to your knee or come as close as possible. Return to your original position and do the same on the opposite side.

JOG PUNCHES

Jogging is a great exercise to get your heart rate up, burn calories, and tone your muscles. This is a perfect HIIT (High Intensity Interval Training) maneuver, as you can alter your running speed according to your level of fitness or goals. To make this exercise even more beneficial and to incorporate more muscle groups into the workout, punching the air while running in place is an easy addition. As with many of these exercises, engage your core to increase abdominal strength and toning. Make sure you breathe smoothly during the exercise and establish a rhythm.

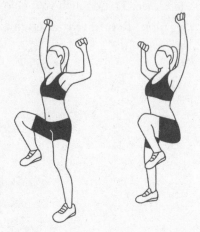

HOW TO

1. Stand with feet shoulder-width apart and arms in a position as if you are about to jog in place.

2. Start running in place, but instead of pumping your arms forward, lift them up and punch them in the air rapidly, alternating between arms.

3. Keep pumping your arms as long as your feet are moving.

4. Perform this exercise by alternating between periods of activity and periods of rest.

Exercise Variation: Instead of running in place, walk quickly in place and pump your arms in the air.

JUMPING JACKS

Jumping jacks are a staple when teaching children exercise for a good reason—they use lots of muscles and activate the cardiovascular system at the same time. Some of the areas whose muscles are sure to get a good workout include: calves, hips, thighs, shoulders, and core. While much of the focus for this 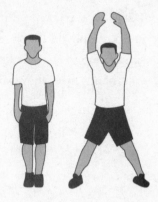 exercise surrounds burning fat and strengthening the heart muscle, which needs to pump vigorously to circulate the oxygenated blood, balance and coordination are enhanced too. When doing the maneuver correctly, your limbs need to be coordinated with your jumps and brain, and this helps develop better posture, rhythm, balance, and timing—all things that we need for other exercises or daily functions of living.

HOW TO

1. Stand upright in a relaxed position with your arms by your sides and feet together.

2. Slightly bend your knees, then jump into the air, making sure both feet get off the ground.

3. While jumping, spread your legs apart and bring your stretched hands up above your head and have them slightly touch or clap at their apex.

4. Jump back to your original position.

5. Repeat.

Exercise Variation: If you have any physical limitations and can't jump, simply do the same hand motion, but instead of jumping, simply step to one side first, then step to the other side next while your hands meet above your head.

WALKING

For many people, getting up out of a chair or off the sofa is a big enough change to actually show both physiologic and aesthetic improvements. Movement is the foundational stimulus to get the heart beating faster and muscles contracting more. Both of these activities will increase the number of calories burned. Walking is a great place to start, and one should never be embarrassed to include it as part of an exercise regimen.

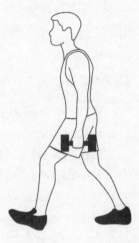

There are all kinds of things you can do to enhance the intensity of your walk as well as the impact it will have on your cardiovascular system and muscle toning and strengthening. Purchase a pair of 3- or 5-pound dumbbells and pump your arms while walking to not only add to the increased cardiac demand, but also to strengthen and tone your upper body. Vary the speed of your walk. Set your stopwatch and walk fast for a designated amount of time, then resume a more casual gait. Alternate these varying periods of intensity and you will reap more benefits.

Investing in a device that will keep track of your steps is definitely beneficial. You can keep track of the steps taken throughout the day, trying your best to meet the goal listed for that day's workout. Many people who start keeping track of their steps find themselves increasingly motivated to make sure they reach or even exceed their goal. Once this happens, you might even set mini goals for yourself such as completing the steps earlier each day or even exceeding the suggested total.

Walking is also something that you can do with others, which makes it less about being a chore and more about spending quality time with someone else as you get your exercise accomplished.

HOW TO

1. Walk at a casual pace with your arms pumping at your side.

2. Walk at a moderate pace with your arms pumping at your side.

3. Fast walk for a specified amount of time, then return back to slow walking, then back to fast walking.

4. Walk with light dumbbells (3 to 5 pounds) in your hands, occasionally doing bicep curls as you walk.

5. As you build your endurance, complete a timed fast walk, looking to improve your time every couple of weeks.

STAR JUMPS

This exercise works your quadriceps femoris (thigh muscles), gastrocnemius muscles (calves), and glutes (buttocks). Star jumps are a good way to increase your endurance, and the explosiveness of the move activates your musculoskeletal system in a way that requires a huge burst of energy, thus increasing your caloric burn. Imagine doing a jumping jack without clapping your hands at the top of the jump.

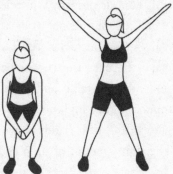

HOW TO

1. Stand upright in a state of relaxation with your feet shoulder-width apart and your arms held closely to your body.

2. Squat down halfway (your buttocks about 6 inches above parallel) and explode upward toward the sky as high as possible.

3. During your upward explosion, extend your body by spreading your arms and legs out as if making the points of a star.

4. Upon landing, bring your arms and legs back in and bend your knees slightly so that your legs absorb the impact.

5. Give yourself a second of rest, regain your form and composure, and jump again.

STEP-UPS

This exercise sounds and looks simple, but there's so much you can get from it. The requirements are easy—the bottom of a staircase or a box made of durable material that can sustain your weight. Doing this exercise properly will primarily work the muscles of your thighs, calves, and buttocks. You can also vary the exercise as you become more comfortable and your balance improves, by raising your opposite knee high once your other foot is solidly on the platform and lifting your hands above your head. Performing step-ups for the right amount of time and the right speed can really get your heart rate going and those calories burning.

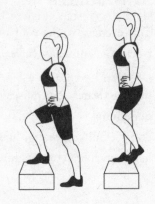

HOW TO

1. Stand in front of a step or a box 12 inches or less in height with your hands hanging by your side.

2. With either your right or left foot, step up onto the top of the stair or box, bringing the other foot alongside it so that both feet are on top together.

3. Whichever foot was used first to initiate the step, step back down with that foot, then bring the other foot to rest beside it on the floor.

4. Repeat this sequence, increasing the speed of the cycle to increase the challenge of the exercise.

Exercise Variation: Hold light dumbbells in your hands while doing the exercise to increase the resistance and thus benefits of the exercise.

STAIRS

One of the best pieces of exercise equipment is sitting right there in your house—flights of stairs. Walking up and down steps is a more demanding exercise than most think. When you're young and well conditioned, you don't give a second thought to climbing or descending a couple of flights of stairs. However, as one ages and becomes deconditioned, serious thought is given to avoiding stairs because of the level of effort required, coordination needed, and physical rigor involved. Use stairs for more than going from one floor to the next, as a no-frills way to challenge your body.

HOW TO

1. When going up steps, focus on stepping and landing on the balls of your feet (front foot pad) when going to the next step.

2. Push your feet into the step and use your thigh muscles and the balls of your feet to spring up.

3. Avoid holding on to the railing if possible, but if you need it for safety measures, by all means do so.

4. Going up one flight and back down a flight is considered to be one set.

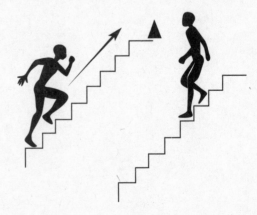

INTERMEDIATE

ICE SKATERS

PLANK

SQUAT JUMPS

LINE HOPS

CYCLING

BUTT KICKS

PLANK JACKS

HIGH KNEES (RUNNING)

LUNGES

MODIFIED GRASSHOPPER

ICE SKATERS

This exercise gives you a lot of return for your investment. Imagine the speed skaters in the Olympics racing down the ice. You are going to simulate their motion, but in a static position rather than moving forward like they do. Form is important when doing this exercise, so keep your upper body slightly bent forward and your head up. Your quads will get a great burn with this exercise and your heart and lungs will also feel the rush.

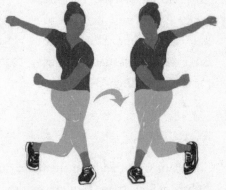

HOW TO

1. Start with your feet a little wider than your shoulders. Looking directly forward, keep your back straight and your knees slightly bent.

2. In one motion, take your right leg and extend it behind you toward the left side of your body so that it is farther left than your left leg; take your left hand and bend it down toward the right side of your body and touch the ground.

3. Next, do the same motion, but switch sides. Bring your right leg back to its starting position and at the same time bring your left leg across behind the right side of your body; at the same time touch the ground in front of your left side with your right hand.

4. Repeat this alternating movement for the desired number of reps.

PLANK

This increasingly popular maneuver is a great addition to anyone looking to strengthen their core and get those pronounced abdominal muscles. Doing this exercise correctly, however, is extremely important for those truly looking to maximize the gains. Perform the exercise for only the length of time that you can remain in proper form. As you become stronger, you will be able to increase the time. Don't rush. This exercise is as meditative as it is strengthening.

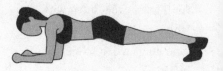

HOW TO

1. Plant your hands on the floor, directly under your shoulders, slightly wider than shoulder-width apart. Pretend that you're about to do a push-up.

2. Press your toes into the ground and tighten your butt muscles (glutes). Make sure you don't lock or hyperextend your knees.

3. Keep your head in line with your back, and neutralize the neck and spine by focusing on a spot on the floor.

4. Hold this position for 15 seconds to start. The more comfortable and better conditioned you are, the longer you can hold the plank.

Exercise Variation: To do a **Forearm Plank**, follow the same instructions as the regular plank, but set your forearms on the ground instead of your hands. Keep your palms flat on the ground in front of you or clasp them together—whichever is comfortable.

Exercise Variation: To do a **Knee Plank**, rest your knees on the ground, with your forearms locked and your hands resting flat on the ground (the same position as for a regular plank). Having the knees on the ground reduces the stress in your lower back.

SQUAT JUMPS

This takes the basic squat that's listed in the previous beginner section of exercises and adds the dimension of a jump. The jumping feature will increase the intensity of muscle engagement, and the added explosiveness along with the landing are important to spike the heart rate and the fast-twitch muscles of the leg. This complex (multi-joint) exercise provides a tremendous workout in a very short period of time.

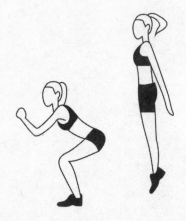

HOW TO

1. Stand up straight with your feet shoulder-width apart and hands by your side.

2. Drop into a squat position and bring your arms up to a 90-degree angle about chest high, with your hands balled into fists or bent into a claw formation. Hold for 3 seconds.

3. Take a deep breath, then in one motion, bring your arms behind you like a pumping mechanism, then explode into the air with your hands helping you thrust upward. Land back in a squat position when you reach the ground.

4. Repeat this sequence.

5. As your stamina builds, increase the number of jumps you do over a specified amount of time.

LINE HOPS

This is one of my favorite exercises, because it requires nothing but a line and determination. Draw a line on the ground or find a line or crack or lay down a string or rope to make the line. Jumping over the line from one side to the other is all the exercise calls for, but it can create a great physical demand when you do it for a concentrated period of time. The beauty of this exercise is that you can do the hops in a variety of forms, whether with both feet, one at a time, or simply stepping over quickly without jumping. Be prepared to work your thigh, calf, and hip muscles.

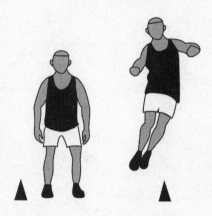

HOW TO

1. Stand with both feet together on one side of a line with your hands by your side bent at a 90-degree angle as if you are about to run.

2. Slightly crouch down, then explode into the air, jumping up and laterally to clear the line with both feet at the same time and land on the other side on the balls of your feet.

3. Once you land, hop right back up and over the line to your original position.

4. Repeat this sequence, continuously jumping from one side to the other without rest.

Exercise Variation: Instead of jumping with both feet, simply place one foot over the line to the other side, and once that lands, bring the other one over quickly. Pump your arms while doing this, bringing your feet back across the line in reverse order. To get your heart rate up, make sure you do this as fast as you can.

CYCLING

There's so much that can be done and said about this exercise. A review of all the variations in equipment and riding strategies would take a chapter of its own. Cycling is a well-known aerobic exercise, but it can also be critical for muscle strengthening and toning. Among the many muscles used are the quadriceps, calf muscles, glutes, hamstrings, hips, and feet. It's important to pick a machine and bike that works well for you. Making the proper adjustments with the seat and pedals is critical, as this can be a very explosive exercise that recruits large muscles and can be stressful on your joints. Paying attention to the ergonomics will pay dividends with regard to safety and efficiency.

HOW TO

1. Sprint as fast as you can for a specified period of time (for example: 35 seconds), then pedal slowly for an equal period of time, then go back to your fast pedal. Alternate this fast and slow pace three or four times.

2. Decide a total distance you wish to travel, then break up the ride into equal segments. Alternate your speed, as well as the resistance you apply, between the segments.

3. Alternate your bike ride with other cardio machines in the gym such as the elliptical or treadmill. Incorporate it into a "cardio threesome" and maximize your caloric burn.

4. Choose a set total distance you wish to accomplish. Every few times you do the bike, try to shave 10% off your time until you're going as fast as you can for that specified distance.

BUTT KICKS

This is meant to be a relatively simple cardiovascular exercise and is often used by runners, basketball players, and tennis players as they warm up before a game or practice. Imagine running in place but adding a new dimension of kicking your legs up behind you so that you softly tap your buttocks. You will be able to work your hamstrings and glutes and stretch your quads, which can unknowingly tighten up throughout the day.

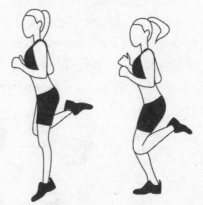

HOW TO

1. Stand erect with your arms by your sides and your feet shoulder-width apart.

2. Move forward by kicking one foot ahead and the other behind you toward your butt.

3. The hand opposite the foot touching your butt is simultaneously raised to your shoulder in a pumping motion.

4. As you lift your heels, your thighs shouldn't move.

5. As you become familiar with the exercise, try to increase your speed and/or duration. If you don't completely touch your butt with your foot, don't worry. Just get it up as high as you can.

PLANK JACKS

This exercise is all about taking planks to the next level. Not only will you be working your core, but you will now put greater emphasis on your upper body, legs, and hip muscles. Form is extremely important for this exercise. To get the best results and to avoid injury, you must make sure you're doing the exercise correctly. The impetus is to lift your butt into the air so that your body is in an upside-down V formation, but this is not correct form. The exercise will be easier to complete, but you will not be maximizing the benefits.

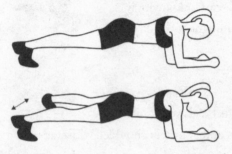

HOW TO

1. Begin in a plank position—shoulders over your wrists, back straight, body in a downward line and feet together. You can also do the position where you rest your forearms on the ground instead of your hands.

2. Imagine doing a jumping jack on the ground. Keep your upper body still while jumping your legs out wide, then back together. Make sure you keep your body's line intact, and don't let your buttocks pop up or your pelvis twist.

3. Decide on a specified number of jumps you want to do per set, then do at least three sets.

HIGH KNEES (RUNNING)

This exercise takes the marching form of high knees to a new level. The muscles that are worked remain the same, but the intensity level is increased dramatically. Instead of marching in place with your knees pumping up and your arms pumping by your side, you will now be running in place while executing the maneuver. The demand on your legs and lungs is quite high, so just a short period of exercise (30 to 45 seconds) can pay big dividends with regard to boosting metabolism and increasing muscle tone.

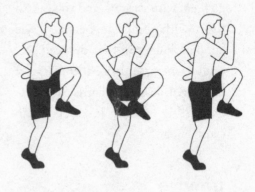

HOW TO

1. Stand straight with your feet apart no wider than your hips. Make sure your arms are hanging down by your sides and your back is straight as you look forward.

2. Jump from one foot to another as if running in place, making sure that you lift your knees as high as possible.

3. Your arms should be bent to 90 degrees with your hands clamped into fists. Pump your arms up and down in the same motion as your legs, which should be pumping up to the height of your waist.

4. Be light on your feet; make sure your heels never strike the ground, but only the balls of your feet as you continue the jumping motion for the duration of the exercise.

LUNGES

Lunges are a great lower extremity–strengthening exercise. When it comes to toning your legs, there aren't many exercises that can match the benefits of a lunge. There are many ways to perform this exercise, and this flexibility allows you to increase or decrease the difficulty of execution. You can do them with weights, and you can do them with jumps in between (see jumping lunges in the advanced section) to increase the challenge. Most important, learn the correct form, as doing this exercise improperly can cause injury.

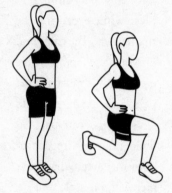

HOW TO

1. Start with your upper body straight and your shoulders held back and relaxed. Keep your chin up and head level.

2. Engage your core and step forward with one leg by lowering your hips until both knees are at a 90-degree angle—the one that is almost touching the ground and the one that is up in the air. Keep the knee that's out front directly above your ankle without pushing it out too far. The knee closer to the ground should come close, but not touch, the ground.

3. Once the lunge is complete, keep the weight in your heels while pushing back up to the starting position.

4. Repeat the sequence, except alternate which leg goes forward and which one goes toward the ground.

5. When you want more of a challenge, do the same maneuver, but instead of standing back up to your original position, walk forward doing sequential lunges. This is a very advanced variation, but excellent at getting your heart rate up and increasing muscle tone.

MODIFIED GRASSHOPPER

This multiphase exercise will work your core, arms, and leg muscles. It might take a few tries to get the movement down correctly, so don't get frustrated and give up. The benefits it delivers are well worth your patience. It's important to keep your abdominal muscles tightened throughout the process for maximal contraction. The faster you go, the greater the cardiovascular workout you will achieve.

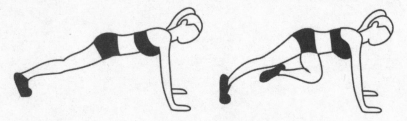

HOW TO

1. Start in push-up position with your hands directly underneath your shoulders.

2. Pull your right leg forward and tuck it sideways while doing so, bringing your knee up and to the left side of your body. (For those doing a full grasshopper, bring your knee all the way forward so that it just touches the inside of your left arm.) Make sure you tighten your core (abdominal muscles) while doing this maneuver. Keep your leg off the ground the entire time.

3. Return your left leg back to starting position, and then bring your right leg forward, tucking it sideways and to the left side of your body. (For those doing a full grasshopper, bring your knee all the way forward so that it just touches the inside of your left arm.) Continue to keep your core tightened and legs off the ground during the maneuver.

4. As you master the exercise, you can do it faster to increase the sustained abdominal contraction and cardiovascular challenge.

ADVANCED

BURPEES

MOUNTAIN CLIMBERS

AB TWISTS

KETTLEBELL SWINGS

ROWING

SPRINTING

TUCK JUMPS

FROG JUMPS

BOX JUMPS

JUMPING LUNGES

BURPEES

This multiphase exercise is a full-body exercise and is great at targeting your core, arms, chest, back, glutes, and legs. Expect a good spike in your heart rate and burn in your muscles. This exercise is most beneficial when you try to complete a certain number of burpees in a specific time. To challenge yourself as you become familiar with the exercise, increase the number of burpees you perform in that same period of time or increase the length of time you do the burpees.

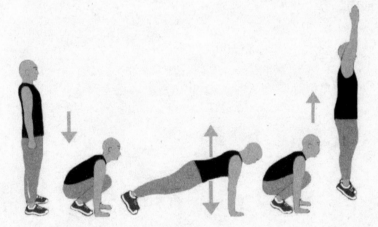

HOW TO

1. Stand with your feet spread hip-width apart and your arms resting down by your sides. Put more of your weight on the front portion of your feet with your heels slightly off the ground.

2. Lower yourself into a squat position, making sure you steady yourself by placing your hands flat on the floor in front of you.

3. Once you reach the squat position and your hands are on the floor, quickly kick your legs backward so that your body is extended into a push-up position.

4. Lower your chest to an inch above the floor just as you would if doing a push-up. Make sure you don't let your chest hit the floor.

5. In one motion, push your chest back up and kick your legs forward so that you're back into a squat position.

6. From the squat position, use your legs to push off the ground and jump as high as you can into the air, then repeat from step 1 again.

MOUNTAIN CLIMBERS

This is a rigorous exercise that can pay dividends immediately. This requires coordination, strength, and endurance, but when done properly, the caloric burn you achieve can be stratospheric. Start by doing small timed intervals, then increase as your endurance builds. This is a full-body exercise that will impact muscles from head to toe.

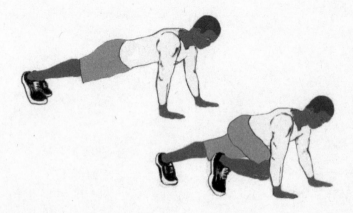

HOW TO

1. Start as if in a push-up position, but with your hands wider than your shoulders and in front. Slightly elevate your buttocks, but not too high. Start with your left foot forward until it comes to rest on the floor under your chest. At this point your left knee and hip are bent, and your thigh is in toward your chest. Your right knee should be off the ground, with your right leg extended straight and strong. Your right toes are tucked under, heel up. Contract your abdominal muscles to stabilize your spine.

2. Keep your hands firmly on the ground, and jump so that you can switch leg positions. Now your left leg is extended straight behind you and your right leg is bent underneath your chest with your right foot on the floor. Be sure to keep your abdominals engaged and shoulders strong. Do not lift your buttocks too high, as that will defeat the purpose of the exercise. Keep your head up and looking forward.

3. Repeat.

AB TWISTS

This exercise is extremely effective at isolating your abdominal muscles and helping you attain that ripped look. You can modify this exercise to make it easier or more challenging. The easier version would allow you to keep your feet on the floor while doing the twist. The more challenging version would call for you to hold weights or a medicine ball while doing the twist. This exercise is accessible to all fitness levels with these modifications.

HOW TO

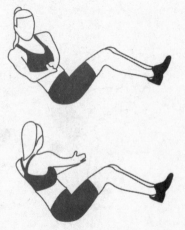

1. Sit on a flat surface with your knees slightly bent.

2. Lean back and lift your legs so that they are about 6 inches off the ground.

3. Keep your back straight while doing the exercise and avoid hunching forward.

4. Swing your left arm and hand across your chest and twist your body to the right. Go back to the beginning position and this time twist your body to the left while bringing your right arm and hand across your chest.

5. Exhale while doing the twisting motion and inhale while returning to center position.

KETTLEBELL SWINGS

This exercise is a great combination of resistance and cardio training. Not only does it increase your heart rate, but it works on strengthening muscles in your shoulders, back, forearms, buttocks, thighs, and calves. Kettlebell swings offer you plenty of options to increase the intensity of your workout, whether it's by using a heavier bell or increasing the number of repetitions. Make this a part of your workout regimen and the results won't disappoint you.

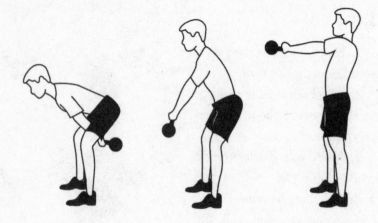

HOW TO

1. Choose a kettlebell that is the right weight (typically 5 to 10 pounds for most people, but more if you're stronger and better conditioned) that allows you to swing with proper technique yet is challenging. You should be able to do 10 consecutive swings with that weight.

2. Stand erect with your feet slightly wider than your shoulders, holding the kettlebell with both hands, palms facing down as they grip the handle. The kettlebell should be held between your legs. Keep your chest up, shoulders back and down, and core engaged.

3. Squat down and bend slightly forward, swinging the kettlebell back between your legs, then once the bell is under your buttocks, drive your feet into the ground and thrust forward with your hips, swinging the bell forward, keeping your arms straight and extended, lifting the bell up to chest level while bringing your body erect again to your starting position.

4. Repeat this sequence for a specified number of repetitions or to complete the exercise in a specified amount of time.

ROWING

The rowing machine might be the best, most underutilized machine in the gym. It provides a full-body workout that is supremely efficient and a mega–calorie burner. When done properly, it works every muscle in the body and creates a calorie burn that continues long after the exercise is over. One of the best ways to use the machine is to alternate it with other machines in the gym such as the treadmill, bicycle, or elliptical. Using the rowing machine properly is important, so make sure a professional shows you how to make the proper adjustments and how to pull the machine correctly to avoid injury and maximize the effectiveness of the workout.

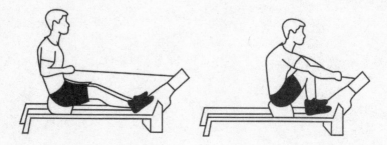

HOW TO

1. Sit tall on the rowing machine seat with your arms straight and holding the handle, back upright, knees and ankles flexed, feet locked onto the angled foot pads.

2. Pull your shoulders down while at the same time tightening your core.

3. Push your legs into the foot pads, moving your body back in the moveable seat until your legs are straightened. While this is happening, lean back to about 45 degrees.

4. Pull the handles toward your torso, but not too high. You should aim for a spot a few inches above your belly button.

5. Finish the exercise maneuver by doing everything in reverse order as you slide back to the original position and the handle and chain are still being held but recoiled back toward the machine.

SPRINTING

Running might be the single most effective way to raise your metabolism, burn fat, increase stamina, and tone your muscles. If you have access to a treadmill, this can help you vary your workout by alternating the speed and incline of your run. However, the beauty of running is that you can have an effective workout even if you don't have a machine. A strip of road or sidewalk or gym is all you need to get out there and shift your metabolism into overdrive. While jogging at a relatively consistent speed over a period of time can be effective at fat burning and weight loss, a program of sprinting interspersed with rest is definitely more productive for the same amount of time.

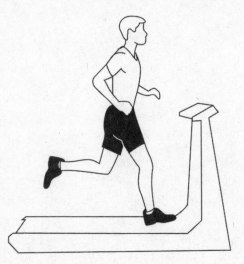

HOW TO (on a treadmill)

1. With your feet off the treadmill belt and on the side of the machine, make sure the incline remains at zero, but increase the speed until you are at an all-out sprint.

2. Safely hop on the moving belt and sprint for 35 seconds.

3. Once the 35 seconds has elapsed, hop off the moving belt and rest for 35 seconds.

4. Repeat this sequence of sprinting and resting.

Exercise Variation: Increase the challenge of this exercise by adding an incline setting on the machine. Try to at least take the incline up to a 2 or 3. The better your condition, the higher you should take up the incline setting.

TUCK JUMPS

Tuck jumps are an explosive full-body-weight exercise that serves double duty as a cardiovascular stimulator and lower-extremity strengthener. Include this in your HIIT routine and you will find that it becomes a valuable calorie burner as it kicks your heart rate into high gear. Form is critical to the success of this exercise. Try jumping as fast as you can without compromising the form.

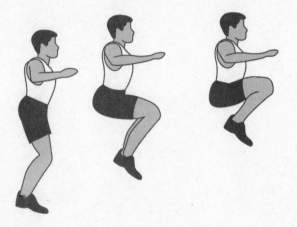

HOW TO

1. Stand straight in a comfortable position with your knees slightly bent and core tightened.

2. Squat a little by dropping your buttocks toward the ground, then jump as high as you can.

3. Tuck your knees together and drive them up toward your chest.

4. Land on your feet with your knees slightly bent to absorb the force as quietly as possible.

5. Repeat this sequence for a set number of jumps or for a specified amount of time.

FROG JUMPS

This plyometric exercise is not for the faint of heart. It not only engages the cardiovascular and muscular systems, but in a very short period of time it can cause a spike in your metabolic demands and thus increase your caloric burn. There are two major variations of the jump, both effective at helping you meet your fitness goals.

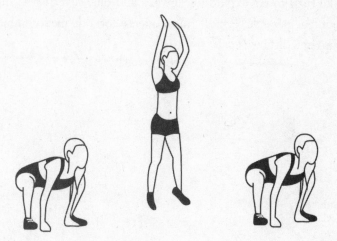

HOW TO

1. Stand in a relaxed position with your feet slightly wider than your shoulders.

2. Drop into a squat position until your thighs are parallel to the ground.

3. Keep your arms in front of you, your elbows inside your knees, your hands slightly resting on the ground.

4. Explode upward into the air while at the same time throwing your hands up.

5. Land as quietly as possible, not on your heels but on the balls of your feet.

Exercise Variation: Instead of squatting and jumping in one place, you can actually perform the exercise with forward movement akin to how a frog would hop and advance at the same time. Perform the same steps above, but instead of exploding upward, make sure you're exploding upward and out, covering as much ground as possible. Repeat this sequence for a defined number of jumps or a distance goal.

BOX JUMPS

It doesn't get much simpler—a box and your legs. If you don't have a box, just use a bench in the park or on a playground. This is a tremendous exercise to increase your leg strength and tone as well as rev up your metabolism so that you burn that unwanted fat. This exercise requires more than just lower-body strength, however. Eye-foot coordination as well as good balance are required to successfully complete this maneuver. Given the heavy demand placed on your lower-extremity muscles and joints, this is not an exercise you want to do on a daily basis, but working it into your routine a couple of times a week can definitely expedite you reaching your fitness goals. Good form with your knees bent and a soft landing will prevent injury.

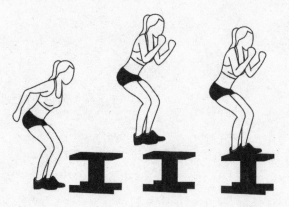

HOW TO

1. Choose a box that fits your physical capabilities (2 to 3 feet). The taller the box, the greater the physical demand to be able to jump safely atop it.

2. Stand in a relaxed position facing the box, knees slightly bent, upper body bent forward slightly on a 45-degree angle and arms bent back against your sides.

3. In the same motion, thrust your arms forward while exploding up into the air and landing on the box with both feet in a squat position and your arms now in front to maintain your balance. Don't land on your heels; rather concentrate on keeping the weight favoring the balls of your feet.

4. Jump back off the box, return to the original position, and repeat.

JUMPING LUNGES

This exercise takes the already demanding lunge to a higher level of difficulty, thus increasing the rewards. This is a great addition to a repertoire of full-body body-weight exercises, as it doesn't require any equipment and can be done anywhere with a small amount of floor space. The benefits are diverse and tangible, engaging a spectrum of muscles, including quads, glutes, hamstrings, calves, hip flexors, hip extensors, and the core. Beyond the muscular engagement, jump lunges also work on balance and coordination, which are requirements to correctly perform this complex exercise.

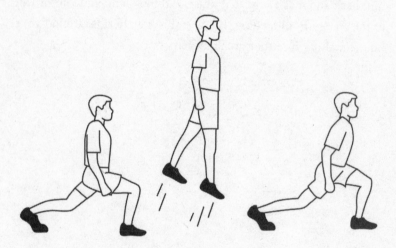

HOW TO

1. Start in a lunge position with one leg forward at a 90-degree angle and one leg back with the knee a few inches above the ground.

2. Hold your arms bent at the elbow at a 90-degree angle with

the arm on the side of the outstretched leg also forward and the other arm back.

3. Lean slightly forward, tighten your core muscles, then quickly sink your weight down, drive both feet into the floor and explode upward in a jump with full extension of your knees and hips so that you look like a diver jumping on a diving board.

4. While in the air and just before landing, switch positions of your feet and arms. The leg and arm that were outstretched before should now be behind you, while the other pair should be forward.

5. Controlling the landing is important, so make sure your forward knee is over your forward foot and not beyond it. Keep your hips back and make sure your knees and hips are bent to absorb all of the energy from landing. Be careful to stay flexible around your knees, making sure they aren't locked.

IV

The EXTRAS

7

CLEAN & LEAN SNACKS

Snacking is an underrated element when it comes to healthy eating and maintaining a balanced meal plan. Snacking is a great way to avoid overindulging when you finally sit down for a full meal. The snacks list below is not meant to be comprehensive but suggestive of the kinds of foods you should choose when trying to satisfy that hunger that slowly creeps in between meals. You can choose to eat from this list or other snacks that meet the clean guidelines. Remember, no artificial ingredients are allowed, as we are avoiding processed foods as much as possible. Are you expected to be perfect? Absolutely not. But should you be able to go thirty days and eat clean snacks 85 percent of the time? Absolutely yes. You know the structure of your daily meal plan, so plan ahead and make sure you have access to clean snacks during the day and at home. If you aren't hungry, then go ahead and skip the snack.

- 1 orange
- 1 apple with almond butter (1 tablespoon)
- Mashed avocado on 100% whole-wheat or whole-grain toast
- 1 cup fresh cherries
- 8-ounce fresh fruit smoothie
- 1 hard-boiled egg with seasoning such as salt and pepper or chile flakes
- 1 cup kale chips (prepared with extra-virgin olive oil)
- 1 cup roasted chickpeas (prepared with extra-virgin olive oil)
- ⅓ cup organic, no-sugar-added trail mix
- ¼ cup unshelled pecans
- 15 walnuts
- 15 cashews
- 20 raw almonds
- ⅓ cup mashed avocado and 8 carrot sticks
- 15 raw or dry-roasted peanuts
- ½ cup black bean dip and 8 veggie sticks (carrots or celery)
- ¾ cup baked apple chips
- ½ cup banana slices and 1 tablespoon organic peanut butter
- 2 slices grilled pineapple
- Fresh fruit popsicle (made only from freshly squeezed juice and frozen into cubes)
- 1 small baked sweet potato
- Small green garden salad

- 1 cup berries
- 1 sliced red pepper with 2 tablespoons hummus
- 10 to 12 baked sweet potato fries brushed with extra-virgin olive oil and sea salt
- 16 baby carrots
- 1 banana
- 10 cherry tomatoes with salt, pepper, and splash of vinaigrette
- ½ cup mushrooms marinated in extra-virgin olive oil, salt, and pepper
- 1 cup watermelon and red onion salad
- 8 watermelon and honeydew melon balls
- ½ cup raw veggies and pesto dip
- 3 cups plain air-popped popcorn
- 1 to 2 cups cucumber and tomato salad with extra-virgin olive oil, salt and pepper to taste
- 15 frozen grapes
- ½ grapefruit
- 4 clean turkey meatballs (1-inch diameter)
- 3 ounces fresh cooked turkey breast slices and ⅓ cup raw veggies or, if deli turkey slices, make sure it's nitrites/nitrates-free, no antibiotics, no artificial flavors, no preservatives
- ⅓ cup pumpkin seeds
- 1 cup mixed fruit salad
- 1 cup shelled edamame
- ½ cup cucumber slices and organic vinaigrette

- 1 large beefsteak tomato slice and 1 tablespoon feta cheese
- ⅔ cup raw veggies and 2 tablespoons guacamole
- 1 apple
- Ten 100% whole-wheat or whole-grain pretzels
- ½ cup organic fat-free or low-fat cottage cheese
- 1 sliced tomato with a pinch of pepper and/or salt and olive oil
- 1 nonfat mozzarella cheese stick with 1 small apple
- ⅓ cup wasabi peas
- 8 to 10 green olives
- ⅓ cup shelled or unshelled sunflower seeds
- 6 ounces organic low-fat or fat-free yogurt with ⅓ cup sliced fruit
- ⅔ cup cauliflower with 2 tablespoons hummus
- 1 celery rib, chopped, with either 2 tablespoons hummus or 2 tablespoons organic peanut butter
- 1 medium apple with 1 tablespoon organic peanut butter
- ⅓ cup egg salad made with clean mayonnaise (see mayonnaise recipe, page 222)
- 7 olives stuffed with 1 tablespoon feta or blue cheese
- 40 raw unsalted pistachios
- 6 watermelon and cucumber skewers on toothpicks with one cube (about the size of one die) feta cheese on each skewer
- ¼ cup (about 20) raw, unsalted mixed nuts
- 20 grapes with 10 almonds or cashews
- 1½ cups sugar snap peas

Homemade Ketchup

2 tablespoons olive oil

1 onion, diced

2 cloves garlic, minced

¼ teaspoon ground allspice

½ teaspoon chili powder

¼ teaspoon powdered ginger

½ teaspoon red pepper flakes

¼ cup apple cider vinegar

¼ cup organic or raw honey

2 tablespoons organic tomato paste or tomato puree

One 28-ounce can peeled whole tomatoes in juice

1 tablespoon organic Worcestershire sauce

¼ teaspoon ground cinnamon

Salt and freshly ground black pepper to taste

1. In a large saucepan, heat the oil and onion over medium-high heat and sauté until translucent, about 8 minutes. Add the garlic, allspice, chili powder, ginger, and red pepper flakes and cook for about 2 minutes.

2. Add the vinegar, honey, tomato paste, tomatoes, Worcestershire sauce, cinnamon, and salt and pepper, then cook for 3 minutes, stirring often.

3. Bring to a slow boil, then lower to a simmer and use a spoon or spatula to crush the whole tomatoes and continue to simmer, uncovered, for 45 to 55 minutes, stirring occasionally, until very thick and smooth. Make sure to keep an eye on it and stir it to keep it from burning.

4. Chill in the refrigerator for at least 1 hour to allow the ketchup to continue thickening and developing flavor.

Clean Mayonnaise

1 large egg

1 egg yolk

½ teaspoon organic
or raw honey

1½ teaspoons fresh lemon juice

1 teaspoon organic mustard

2 teaspoons apple cider vinegar

½ teaspoon salt, plus more
to taste

1 cup extra-virgin olive oil
(this makes the finished
product a little heavier, but
we need to use a clean
ingredient)

If using a mixing bowl:

1. In a medium bowl, combine the egg, egg yolk, honey, lemon juice, mustard, vinegar, and ½ teaspoon salt. Whisk until blended and thickened, 30 to 60 seconds. It should be a bright yellow.

2. In a very slow, steady stream, pour in ½ cup of the oil, whisking continuously, 3 to 5 minutes. Gradually add the remaining ½ cup oil, whisking continuously until the mayonnaise is thickened, about 6 minutes. Now the mayonnaise will appear lighter in color. Season with more salt if needed. Place in an airtight container and keep refrigerated.

If using a blender:

1. Put the egg, egg yolk, honey, lemon juice, mustard, vinegar, and ½ teaspoon salt in a blender. Turn on the blender, then slowly pour the oil in through the hole in the lid a drop at a time, then pour in a thin, slow stream. Blend until the mixture thickens.

2. Taste and adjust your seasoning accordingly.

3. Refrigerate in an airtight container.

Orange-Raspberry Vinaigrette

½ cup freshly squeezed orange juice

¼ cup organic raspberry white balsamic vinegar

2 tablespoons extra-virgin olive oil

1 teaspoon chopped fresh cilantro leaves

Salt and freshly ground black pepper to taste

In a small bowl, whisk together the orange juice, vinegar, oil, and cilantro. Season with salt and pepper. Store in an airtight container in the refrigerator.

Honey Balsamic Vinaigrette

½ teaspoon minced fresh
  basil leaves

1 tablespoon organic
  or raw honey

1 cup extra-virgin olive oil

¼ teaspoon dried oregano

½ teaspoon dried rosemary

⅓ cup white balsamic vinegar

Salt and freshly ground black
  pepper to taste

In a small bowl, whisk together the basil, honey, oil, oregano, rosemary, and vinegar. Season with salt and pepper. Store in an airtight container in the refrigerator.

Quick Salsa Fresca

Nothing comes alive in your mouth like a fresh salsa powered by tomatoes, peppers, garlic, and cilantro. While salsa is a great pairing with chips, it also goes easily with chicken, fish, and pasta. Salsa recipes should be treated like a blueprint created in pencil. Erase whatever you want and add seasonings and vegetables that suit your taste!

Be careful handling the peppers. Wash your hands immediately after with soap and water and don't touch your face or eyes to avoid irritation.

Makes 2 to 3 cups

3 tablespoons finely chopped red onion

2 small cloves garlic, minced

3 cups boiling water

3 large ripe tomatoes, peeled, seeded, and chopped

2 chile peppers (mild or hot)

2 tablespoons minced fresh cilantro (or flat-leaf parsley)

2 tablespoons fresh lime juice

Pinch of ground cumin

Pinch of dried oregano

3 tablespoons cooked black beans (optional)

Salt and freshly ground black pepper to taste

1. Put the onion and garlic in a fine-mesh strainer; 1 cup at a time, pour boiling water over them, then let drain.

2. Once the onion and garlic have cooled, combine them in a medium bowl with the tomatoes, peppers, cilantro, lime juice, cumin, oregano, and beans (if using). Season with salt and black pepper.

3. Refrigerate for 1 to 2 hours to let the flavors blend and settle. This can be refrigerated for up to 1 week. If the salsa is too hot, add more tomatoes to lower the temperature.

INDEX

INDEX

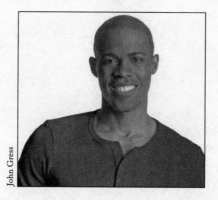

John Gress

IAN K. SMITH, M.D., is the #1 *New York Times* bestselling author of *The Clean 20, SHRED, SUPER SHRED, The SHRED Power Cleanse,* and *Blast the Sugar Out!* He created two national health initiatives—the 50 Million Pound Challenge and the Makeover Mile—and served two terms on President Obama's Council on Fitness, Sports, and Nutrition. A graduate of Harvard, Columbia, and the University of Chicago's Pritzker School of Medicine, Smith is an avid fitness enthusiast and sportsman.

www.shredlife.com
SHREDDER Nation on Facebook
@DrIanSmith on Twitter
@DoctorIanSmith on Instagram